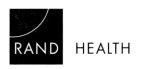
RAND HEALTH

REDIRECTING INNOVATION IN U.S. HEALTH CARE

Options to Decrease Spending and Increase Value

Steven Garber | Susan M. Gates
Emmett B. Keeler | Mary E. Vaiana | Andrew W. Mulcahy
Christopher Lau | Arthur L. Kellermann

The research described in this report was supported by a grant from the Bill & Melinda Gates Foundation and was conducted in RAND Health, a division of the RAND Corporation.

Library of Congress Cataloging-in-Publication Data is available for this publication.

ISBN: 978-0-8330-8546-7

The RAND Corporation is a nonprofit institution that helps improve policy and decisionmaking through research and analysis. RAND's publications do not necessarily reflect the opinions of its research clients and sponsors.

Support RAND—make a tax-deductible charitable contribution at www.rand.org/giving/contribute.html

RAND® is a registered trademark.

Preface

The United States spends more money on health care than any other nation. Many experts identify costly new technology as the biggest driver of health care spending. Previous studies aimed at reining in spending on technology have considered changing how existing medical technologies are used. In contrast, this study focused on changing which medical products get invented in the first place. The goals were to encourage creation of medical products that could improve health and reduce spending or that provide large enough health benefits to warrant any extra spending. The study argues that the most powerful way to accomplish these goals is to realign the financial incentives of inventors, investors, payers, providers, and patients by changing the costs, risks, and rewards anticipated at various stages along the pathway from invention of a medical product to its adoption in the U.S. market. The study suggests policy options that could point the way toward achieving that realignment.

The study should be of interest to health care industry experts, drug and device inventors, regulators, payers and insurers, venture capitalists, health policy experts, legislators, and researchers.

This work was supported by a grant from the Bill & Melinda Gates Foundation. The research was conducted in RAND Health, a division of the RAND Corporation. A profile of RAND Health, abstracts of its publications, and ordering information can be found at www.rand.org/health.

Contents

Figures

Summary

The United States spends more money on health care than any other nation—in total, per capita, and as a percentage of our gross domestic product. Public spending on health care—primarily through the Medicare and Medicaid programs—is crowding out spending on other state and national priorities, including education, Social Security, national defense, and deficit reduction. Private spending on health care takes large bites out of the disposable incomes of U.S. families.

A leading cause of high and growing spending is new medical technologies. Previous studies aimed at reining in spending considered changing the ways in which existing technologies are used. Our work for this project focused on identifying promising policy options to change which medical technologies are created in the first place, with these two related policy goals:

1. Reduce total health care spending with the smallest possible loss of health benefits.
2. Ensure that new medical products that increase spending are accompanied by health benefits that are worth the spending increases.

These goals reflect our definition of the "value" of a medical technology, which compares the increase in population health from using it to the extra spending attributable to its use. A medical product can have large health benefits for some patients and little or no benefit for others. Thus, a key issue for increasing value is improving the alignment between products and patients who will benefit from them.

We define *medical technology* broadly to include all applications of knowledge to practical medical problems. However, in this study we focused more narrowly on *medical products*, specifically drugs, devices, and health information technology (HIT).

To identify promising policy options, we first

- explored how the current U.S. health care system rewards inventors and their private investors for creating and commercializing products that tend to increase health care spending even if they do not provide health benefits that are worth that extra spending

- determined why new medical products that could substantially reduce health care spending often fail to gain traction in U.S. markets.

We argue that the best way to further our twin policy goals is by altering the financial incentives of inventors, private investors, payers, providers, and patients.

Our analysis synthesized information from peer-reviewed and other literature, a panel of technical advisors that was convened for the project, and 50 one-on-one expert interviews. These 30- to 60-minute interviews drew on the experts' firsthand knowledge to gather information about the determinants of medical product invention and adoption. The interview subjects included health care industry experts, drug and device inventors, regulators, payers and insurers, venture capitalists, health policy experts, and researchers.

We also conducted case studies of eight medical products: three drugs (including one biologic), three devices (a diagnostic, an implantable, and a costly machine), and two types of HIT (electronic health records [EHRs] and telemedicine). We use information from the case studies solely for illustrative purposes.

The Context for Medical Product Innovation in the United States

We conceptualize the health care innovation pathway as having three stages:

1. creation of new products, which we call "invention"
2. regulatory approval for sale in the United States
3. processes that determine how and for which patients medical products are used, which we call "adoption."

We highlight what appear to be the most important decisions that determine which products are invented and brought to the U.S. market; the prices charged for them; the coverage, payment, and utilization management policies governing them; which products are used for which patients; and how the new products affect health and spending.

Invention of Medical Products

Inventors include *drug, device, and HIT companies,* and private *investors* provide money to support their inventive efforts. Their decisions about what kinds of products to attempt to create are driven by two key considerations. First, can a potential new product be successfully brought to market? Second, are the expected market rewards large enough to justify the invention and approval costs and risks? Private investors are likely to fund product-invention efforts only if the required investment is likely to generate a healthy financial return, regardless of the product's potential health benefits.

Regulatory Approval of Medical Products

The U.S. Food and Drug Administration (FDA) ultimately decides which products will reach the U.S. market and with what approved uses ("indications"). Its mandate is to ensure that products sold in the United States are safe and effective; doing so can take years. FDA decisions involve major stakes for medical product companies—not only whether products are approved but also how long the review and approval processes take.

Adoption of Medical Products

Providers, such as *hospitals and physicians*, decide which drugs and devices to use and for which patients, as well as which EHR systems to purchase. Many entities try to influence their decisions. *Drug and device manufacturers* directly market their products to prescribers, facilities, and patients. EHR vendors market their products to hospitals and physicians. *Patients* try to influence physician decisions, with limited success. *Public and private payers* influence provider decisions by deciding which products and services will be covered for which patients, how much to pay for covered products and services, and how to promote compliance with their coverage and payment policies.

Thematic Analysis

To help us develop policy options, we distilled five themes from the information we synthesized:

- lack of basic scientific knowledge
- costs and risks of FDA approval
- limited rewards for medical products that could lower spending
- treatment creep
- the medical arms race.

The themes are features of the U.S. health care environment that substantially affect the costs and risks of, and financial rewards for, medical product invention. The first two themes relate to whether a product can be brought to market and the costs and risks of doing so—that is, they relate to the invention and regulatory approval stages of the innovation pathway. The last three themes relate to the adoption stage and describe features of medical product markets that either (1) limit the market rewards that inventors and investors expect from products that could lower spending or otherwise provide good value or (2) provide large market rewards for products that provide low value.

Lack of Basic Scientific Knowledge

Efforts to invent technologies to treat, cure, or prevent a disease are unlikely to progress unless the underlying disease processes are reasonably well understood. Many high-burden medical conditions lack effective treatments because scientific understanding falls short of what inventors and investors think is sufficient to justify investments. The probabilities of inventing products that are safe and effective figure prominently in the decisions of drug and device inventors and private investors.

Costs and Risks of FDA Approval

Some stakeholders say that FDA approval takes too long, costs too much, and discourages innovation. Others say that the time involved in FDA reviews and approvals is necessary to ensure product safety and effectiveness. Whether or not the regulatory process could be faster without compromising safety, inventors face the following facts: As the time required for approval increases, so do inventors' costs, and so does the time inventors have to wait to generate sales in the United States.

Limited Rewards for Medical Products That Lower Spending

In most U.S. industries, consumers benefit from competition because competitors vie for business by offering product improvements, lower prices, or both. Customers tend to buy from the sellers that provide the best value. Price competition in many U.S. health care markets is not as vigorous as in many other industries, and, as a result, it fails to adequately reward innovators that develop technologies with the potential to lower spending. This failure results from three phenomena:

1. **Limited price sensitivity on the part of consumers and payers:** Key sources of limited price sensitivity include fee-for-service (FFS) payment arrangements that reward providers for providing more care, generously insured patients, lack of price transparency, and limitations on Medicare's ability to consider cost in coverage and payment decisions. Several ongoing trends and developments appear to be increasing price sensitivity. These include increased use of payment methods that put providers at financial risk, increasing deductibles in many private insurance plans, declining prevalence (and generosity) of employer-sponsored health insurance, the excise tax instituted by the Affordable Care Act (ACA) on especially generous employer-sponsored insurance plans (sometimes called "Cadillac plans"), and high cost-sharing rates in the lower-premium plans offered on the health insurance exchanges instituted by the ACA.

2. **The limited time horizon of providers when they decide which medical products to use for which patients:** In many instances, the health benefits from using a drug, device, or HIT are not realized until years in the future, at which time the patient is likely to be covered by a different insurer, such as

Medicare. When this is the case, only the later insurer will obtain the financial benefits associated with the (long-delayed) health benefits.

3. **Fragmented decisionmaking:** Many provider systems are siloed. When this is the case, most decisionmakers consider only the costs and benefits for their parts of their organizations, and few take into account savings that accrue outside of their silos.

Treatment Creep

The value of a treatment or diagnostic test depends on the health benefits it provides for the patients who use it. Undesirable treatment creep often occurs when a medical product that provides substantial benefits to some patients is used for other patients for whom the health benefits are much smaller or completely absent. Treatment creep is encouraged by FFS payment arrangements, and it is enabled by lack of knowledge about which patients would truly benefit from which products. Treatment creep often involves using products for indications not approved by the FDA. Such "off-label" use—which delivers good value in some instances—is widespread and difficult to control. Treatment creep may reward developers with additional profits for inventing products whose use can be expanded to groups of patients who will benefit little.

Medical Arms Race

The "medical arms race" refers to hospitals and other facilities competing for business by making themselves attractive to physicians, who may care more about using new high-tech services than they care about lower prices. Many patients also prefer the latest, high-tech treatments. Because hospitals want to keep equipment operating near capacity in order to recoup its costs—and physicians make money by helping them do so—providers often use expensive technologies for patients for whom the health benefits are small. Robotic surgery for prostate cancer and proton beam radiation therapy provide striking examples of undesirable treatment creep: Although there is little or no evidence that they are superior to traditional treatments, these high-cost technologies have been successfully marketed directly to patients, hospitals, and physicians. High market rewards for such expensive technologies encourage inventors and investors to develop more of them—regardless of how much they improve health.

Options to Reduce Costs and Risks of Invention and Approval

Using perspectives suggested by the innovation pathway, literature, our interviewees, and a panel of experts convened for the project, we developed ten high-priority policy options. These are the options that we think are most promising in terms of advancing our two policy goals, based on all of our sources of information and our judgment about which of the many options that we considered are most likely to have major impact. We first present five options for encouraging the invention of drugs and devices that would further our policy goals by reducing the costs and/or risks of invention and obtaining FDA approval:

1.   Enable more creativity in funding basic science.
2.   Offer prizes for inventions.
3.   Buy out patents.
4.   Establish a public-interest investment fund.
5.   Expedite FDA reviews and approvals.

Enable More Creativity in Funding Basic Science

Invention of new medical technologies typically builds on a base of basic biomedical science. Major breakthroughs in medical product development often require earlier breakthroughs in basic science, which likely require many scientists to pursue innovative and risky research programs. For the most part, however, the National Institutes of Health (NIH), the largest federal investor in biomedical research, relies on methods for choosing and funding research that favor low-risk projects, and if investigators fail to achieve their project goals, future NIH funding becomes less likely. A different model is used by the Howard Hughes Medical Institute, which funds scientists rather than projects, encourages risk-taking, and seems more willing than NIH is to provide additional funding to scientists whose past risky endeavors did not pan out.

Offer Prizes for Inventions

Substantial "prizes" could be awarded to the first individuals or groups that invent drugs or devices that satisfy prespecified criteria relating to their performance. Prizes could be offered by such public entities as the Centers for Medicare & Medicaid Services (CMS) or NIH, by private health care systems, by philanthropists and charitable foundations, or by public-private partnerships. An intriguing alternative to an immediate cash payment is a share of future savings to the Medicare program that could be attributed to an invention.

Buy Out Patents

Purchasing patents on products that have already been invented could increase rewards for inventing products that could decrease spending but are financially unattractive to inventors and investors. Public agencies, private philanthropists, or public-private partnerships might purchase patents. The purpose would be to ensure that a product is commercialized and offered at low prices. A purchaser could (1) put the patent in the public domain, and offerings by several manufacturers could then generate price competition, or (2) license the technology selectively, specifying the highest price that licensees could charge for the product. Realistically, only a small number of patents could be purchased if purchasing required full payment up front, so purchasers would need to be very selective. As with prizes, however, the best approach might be to offer patent holders a share of the savings to the Medicare program that could be attributed to the patented inventions.

Establish a Public-Interest Investment Fund

The market rewards for inventing products that reduce spending are often too low to be attractive to private investors. A public-interest investment fund (PIIF) could finance such inventive efforts. Such a fund would require both initial and ongoing investment capital.

Rather than relying on government officials to "pick winners," it would be very desirable to tap the expertise of experienced private-sector investors. A private-public partnership might be the best approach for doing so. For example, private investors could be motivated to help make the investment decisions by being allowed to invest in projects supported by the fund, with a share of Medicare savings offered to make potential returns attractive to them.

Expedite FDA Reviews and Approvals for Technologies That Decrease Spending

Review and approval processes could be speeded up, but not watered down, for medical products that are expected to substantially reduce spending. Four mechanisms already exist to speed FDA review and approval. However, criteria for which drugs and devices can use these mechanisms involve only health effects—e.g., a product will fill an unmet need for a serious condition. Creating a mechanism to expedite reviews for products expected to reduce spending could lower inventors' regulatory costs for such products. Creating the mechanism would require new legislation to expand the FDA's mission to include spending.

Policy Options to Increase Market Rewards

We also present five options for encouraging the invention of drugs and devices that would further our two policy goals by increasing market rewards.

1. Reform Medicare payment policies.
2. Reform Medicare coverage policies.
3. Coordinate FDA approval and CMS coverage processes.
4. Increase demand for technologies that decrease spending.
5. Produce more and more-timely technology assessments.

Reform Medicare Payment Policies

If CMS were allowed to consider cost in determining payment rates—which would require new legislation—the agency could set Medicare rates to save money in the short run and improve inventors' incentives over the long run.

One widely discussed possibility is for Medicare to move more quickly away from FFS payment approaches and toward approaches that reduce financial rewards to providers when spending is higher than needed to deliver quality care. Such approaches include *bundled payment* for episodes of care and *capitated* arrangements that provide fixed payments per person to provide all covered care. Expanding the use of such payment approaches—CMS already uses prospective payment approaches for hospital stays outpatient procedures—would put providers at financial risk for low-value care in additional circumstances and thereby increase their demand for less costly approaches to care. In turn, this could increase demand for medical products that would decrease spending.

Reform Medicare Coverage Policies

CMS could change its coverage determination policies in ways that would increase the health benefits per dollar of Medicare spending. We suggest several potential reforms, some of which would require new legislation. For example, CMS could expand use of its existing "coverage with evidence" process. Medicare could also stop paying for tests, procedures, and technologies that clinical experts have deemed inappropriate or ineffective; many of these have already been identified by the Choosing Wisely initiative. Medicare could also stop covering off-label use of some very expensive cancer and other specialty drugs in circumstances in which there is little or no evidence of effectiveness—a reform that would require new legislation.

Coordinate FDA Approval and CMS Coverage Processes

Another potential way to stimulate invention of products that decrease spending is to coordinate CMS coverage and payment determination processes with FDA review and approval processes. This could involve, for example, concurrent reviews, with CMS specifying early in the FDA review process what evidence CMS requires in addition to that required by the FDA. NIH scientists might also be involved as experts.

Coordination could reduce the time required to move a product to market. This option could be viewed as an extension of the FDA's Innovation Pathway 2.0 initiative. Identifying the best approach might be informed, for example, by what is learned from existing efforts involving parallel review by FDA and CMS. The Office of the Secretary of the U.S. Department of Health and Human Services would be an appropriate venue for considering the potential for coordination, the pros and cons of different approaches, and specifying new requirements and rules.

Increase Demand for Technologies That Decrease Spending

Changing payer, provider, and patient incentives could increase demand for products that seem likely to help reduce spending. An across-the-board increase in cost-sharing or increasing use of high-deductible health plans could lead patients to request low-cost services or reject physician recommendations for high-cost ones. However, across-the-board increases in cost-sharing are undesirable because they undermine the financial risk–pooling function of insurance, and patients are likely to cut back on both low- and high-value care in response.

A more promising alternative is expanding use of value-based insurance designs (VBIDs), which require patients to pay more out of pocket to receive low-value services than for high-value ones. A key challenge for VBID, as for other policy options we have mentioned, is determining whether a service has high or low value for individual patients. This leads to our last policy option.

Produce More and More-Timely Technology Assessments

Health technology assessments (HTAs)—comparative effectiveness and cost-effectiveness analyses, for example—provide systematic evidence about the safety, efficacy, effectiveness, and cost of drugs, devices, and procedures. Such evidence can help payers and providers predict which patients are likely to benefit substantially from a technology's use. HTAs are conducted by both public entities and private organizations. Some of the latter share their assessments at no charge, while others do not. Medical technology evolves quickly, and thus HTAs are more useful when they are more current. Much more will be learned in the coming years about the comparative effectiveness of many medical interventions through research supported by the Patient Centered Outcomes Research Institute (PCORI). A provision of the Affordable Care Act, however, greatly limits consideration of costs in research supported by PCORI.

There is an emerging commercial model for producing more-timely HTAs. Specifically, rather than spending years to produce an HTA and updating it only years later if at all, a commercial entity called UpToDate keeps abreast of the literature via frequent literature searches and revises its HTAs whenever new findings warrant.

Concluding Thoughts

The rate of growth of U.S. spending on health care appears to have declined in recent years, and some ongoing trends will help reduce spending. The facts remain, however, that spending on health care in the United States constrains our opportunities to make progress on major public and private priorities other than health, and there is substantial room for reducing spending in ways requiring only fairly small sacrifices in population health.

Because the stakes in reining in health care spending and getting more health benefits from the money we do spend are so high, we believe that all promising options should be considered—*and the sooner the better*. However, as helpful as it may be to change the nature of future drugs and devices, we cannot reasonably expect our two policy goals to be adequately addressed only by changing the incentives of inventors. For example, much of our health care spending does not involve drugs or devices.

Various stakeholders can be expected to resist many of these policy options. Fundamentally reforming Medicare would likely meet the most powerful resistance. Much of the resistance will decry "rationing" and invoke "rights" of access to health care. Indeed, implementing some or all of our policy options would deny some U.S. residents medical care that would benefit them. However, because it is often the case that people other than the patient are paying the bills, it might be appropriate to conceive of consumer "rights" as pertaining not to all desired health care—effective or not, shockingly expensive or not—but rather only to effective and high-value care.

The longer we wait to institute fundamental reforms, the more money we will spend on health care offering little or no health benefit—and the harder it will be to achieve other major social priorities.

Acknowledgments

The authors are grateful to many individuals who contributed to the research reported here.

We are indebted to the members of the technical advisory panel (TEP) convened for this project for providing information and offering sage advice. The 20 members of the TEP are listed in Chapter Three of the report.

We thank our three technical/peer reviewers, all of whom provided extensive, thoughtful, and constructive comments on the draft final report: Ateev Mehrotra, M.D., M.P.H., M.Sc. (RAND); Joseph P. Newhouse, Ph.D. (Harvard University); and Sara Rosenbaum, J.D. (George Washington University).

We thank the physician authors of the detailed case studies available at www.rand.org/t/RR308: Jonathan Bergman, M.D., M.P.H. (prostate-specific antigen and robotic surgery); Enesha Cobb, M.D., M.T.S., M.Sc. (electronic health records); Nihar R. Desai, M.D., M.P.H. (cardiovascular polypill); Hiu-Fai Fong, M.D. (telemedicine); Benjamin R. Roman, M.D. (Avastin for metastatic breast cancer); Kori Sauser, M.D., M.Sc. (electronic health records); Charles D. Scales, Jr., M.D. (prostate-specific antigen and robotic surgery); Erica S. Spatz, M.D., M.H.S. (implantable cardioverter-defibrillators); and Ashaunta Tumblin, M.D. (*Haemophilus influenzae* type b vaccine).

We are grateful to the following interviewees who have granted permission for us to thank them publicly:

- Goran Ando, M.D.
  Chairman, Novo Nordisk AS
- Paul S. Auerbach, M.D., M.S.
  Redlich Family Professor of Surgery, Division of Emergency Medicine, Stanford University School of Medicine
- Robert Berenson, M.D.
  Institute Fellow, the Urban Institute
- Edmund Billings, M.D.
  Chief Medical Officer, Medsphere

- Philippe Chambon M.D., Ph.D.
  Managing Director, New Leaf Venture Partners LLC
- Peter B. Corr, Ph.D.
  Co-Founder and Managing General Partner, Auven Therapeutics
- Denis A. Cortese, M.D.
  Arizona State University (ASU) Foundation Professor and Director of the ASU Healthcare Delivery and Policy Program, Emeritus President/CEO of Mayo Clinic
- Helen Darling, M.A.
  President and CEO, National Business Group on Health
- David T. Feinberg, M.D., M.B.A.
  UCLA Health
- A. Mark Fendrick, M.D.
  University of Michigan
- Atul Gawande, M.D., M.P.H.
  Surgeon, Brigham and Women's Hospital
  Director, Ariadne Labs
  Professor, Harvard School of Public Health and Harvard Medical School
- Jessica Grossman, M.D.
  President and CEO, Sense4Baby, Inc.
- John D. Halamka, M.D.
  Beth Israel Deaconess Medical Center, Boston, Massachusetts
- Jonathan Hare
  Founder/Executive Chairman, Resilient Network Systems
- William A. Hawkins
  President and CEO, Immucor
- Matt Hermann
  Ascension Ventures
- Michael M. E. Johns, M.D.
  Professor, Schools of Medicine and Public Health
  Emory University
- Allen Kamer
  Co-Founder, Humedica, Inc.
- Karen Katen
  Senior Advisor, Essex Woodlands
- Mohit Kaushal, M.D.
- Curtis T. Keith, Ph.D.
  Chief Scientific Officer, Blavatnik Biomedical Accelerator at Harvard University

- Larry Kessler, Sc.D.
  Professor and Chair, Department of Health Services
  School of Public Health, University of Washington
- Darrell G. Kirch, M.D.
  Association of American Medical Colleges
- Kenneth W. Kizer, M.D., M.P.H.
  Distinguished Professor, University of California Davis (UC Davis) School of Medicine and Betty Irene Moore School of Nursing
  and Director, Institute for Population Health Improvement, UC Davis Health System
- Jacqueline Kosecoff, Ph.D.
  Managing Partner, Moriah Partners
- Harlan M. Krumholz, M.D., S.M.
  Section of Cardiovascular Medicine and the Robert Wood Johnson Foundation Clinical Scholars Program, Department of Internal Medicine, Yale University School of Medicine; Department of Health Policy and Management, Yale School of Public Health; Center for Outcomes Research and Evaluation, Yale–New Haven Hospital, New Haven, Connecticut
- David Lansky, Ph.D.
  President and CEO of PBGH
- Stanley N. Lapidus
  President and CEO of SynapDx Corp.
- Frank Litvack, M.D., F.A.C.C., Los Angeles, California
- Mark S. Litwin, M.D., M.P.H.
  Professor and Chair, Department of Urology
  David Geffen School of Medicine at the University of California, Los Angeles (UCLA)
  Professor of Health Policy & Management, UCLA Fielding School of Public Health
- Thomas Rockwell Mackie, Ph.D.
  Morgridge Institute for Research, University of Wisconsin, Madison
- Arnold Milstein, M.D.
  Professor of Medicine
  Clinical Excellence Research Center Director
  Stanford University
- Eric M. Nelson, Ph.D.
  Biotechnology Business Development Consultant, Chapel Hill, North Carolina
- Peter Neumann, Sc.D.
  Director, Center for the Evaluation of Value and Risk in Health
  Institute for Clinical Research and Health Policy Studies
  Tufts Medical Center

- James Niedel, M.D., Ph.D.
  New Leaf Venture Partners
- Christopher Parks
  Founder and Chief Development Office of Change Healthcare Corp
- James C. Robinson
  Leonard D. Schaeffer Professor of Health Economics
  Director, Berkeley Center for Health Technology
  University of California, Berkeley
- John J. Rydzewski
  Executive Chairman, Enumeral Biomedical Corp.
- David Singer
  Maverick Capital
- Glenn Steele, Jr., M.D., Ph.D.
  President and Chief Executive Officer, Geisinger Health System
- Reed V. Tuckson, M.D., F.A.C.P.
  Managing Director, Tuckson Health Connections, LLC
- Nicholas J. Valeriani
  Chief Executive, West Health
  Professor Sir Nicholas Wald, F.R.S., F.R.C.P.
  Wolfson Institute of Preventive Medicine, Barts and The London School of
  Medicine and Dentistry, Queen Mary University of London
- Mary Woolley
  President and CEO, Research!America

Many RAND colleagues contributed to the research and report in a variety of ways. Jeffrey Wasserman helped us improve the analysis through his participation in several brainstorming sessions. Lauren Andrews scheduled and took notes during most of our expert interviews; others who helped with the interviews included Racine Harris, Sarah Kups, and Michael Zaydman. Maggie Snyder, Toni Christopher, Ingrid Maples, and Tricia Soto provided outstanding administrative support. Our production editor, Jocelyn Lofstrom, kept the process running smoothly, and Nora Spiering did excellent work editing two drafts and the final manuscript under tight deadlines.

All opinions and views expressed in this report are those of the authors and do not necessarily reflect the views of the project sponsor, TEP members, RAND, RAND Health, or their sponsors. Arthur L. Kellermann contributed to this report while he was an employee of the RAND Corporation; the views expressed do not necessarily represent those of the Uniformed Services University of the Health Sciences (Dr. Kellermann's current employer) or the Department of Defense.

Abbreviations

ABIM Foundation	American Board of Internal Medicine Foundation
ACA	Affordable Care Act
ACO	accountable care organization
ARPA-E	Advanced Research Projects Agency—Energy
CBO	Congressional Budget Office
CDC	Centers for Disease Control and Prevention
CEA	cost-effectiveness analysis
CMS	Centers for Medicare & Medicaid Services
COV	coverage expert
CT	computed tomography
DC	direct current
DEV	device inventor
DRG	diagnostic related group
DRUG	drug inventor
EHR	electronic health record
ESI	employer-sponsored insurance
FDA	U.S. Food and Drug Administration
FFS	fee-for-service
GAO	U.S. Government Accountability Office
GDP	gross domestic product
GENX	general health care policy expert
HDHP	high-deductible health plan
HHMI	Howard Hughes Medical Institute

HHS	U.S. Department of Health and Human Services
Hib	*Haemophilus influenzae* type b
HIT	health information technology
HITECH	Health Information Technology for Economic and Clinical Health
HMO	health maintenance organization
HTA	health technology assessment
ICD	implantable cardioverter-defibrillator
ICER	incremental cost-effectiveness ratio
INVES	private investor
IOM	Institute of Medicine
IT	information technology
MRI	magnetic resonance imaging
MU	meaningful use
NICHD	Eunice Kennedy Shriver National Institute of Child Health and Human Development
NIH	National Institutes of Health
ODAC	Oncologic Drugs Advisory Committee Clinical
ONC	Office of the National Coordinator for Health Information Technology
PBM	pharmacy benefit management company
PBRT	proton beam radiation therapy
PCORI	Patient Centered Outcomes Research Institute
PET	positron-emission tomography
PIIF	public-interest investment fund
PROV	provider
PSA	prostate-specific antigen
QALY	quality-adjusted life year
R&D	research and development
RCT	randomized controlled trial
SCD	sudden cardiac death

TEP	technical expert panel
USPTO	U.S. Patent and Trademark Office
VA	U.S. Department of Veterans Affairs
VBID	value-based insurance design
VistA	Veterans' Health Information Systems and Technology Architecture

CHAPTER ONE

Introduction

New medical products, such as novel drugs and devices, and health information technology (HIT) have transformed American medicine—often for the better, but sometimes for the worse. In the United States, the benefits of new medical technology are widely assumed to be worth the associated increase in costs, on average, over all technologies and over all patients for whom they are used. However, this is not true for some technologies, nor is it true for how some technologies are used. The Institute of Medicine (IOM), among other groups, has noted that what Americans get for their health care dollar often falls short of its potential (IOM, 2013).

The United States spends more money on health than any other nation, whether measured in terms of total spending ($2.8 trillion in 2012), spending per capita ($8,915 in 2012), or spending as a percentage of gross domestic product (GDP; 17.2 percent in 2012) (CMS, undated [b]). Growth in health care spending outpaced GDP growth by an average of 2.0 to 2.3 percentage points per year from 1950 to the onset of the Great Recession that began in 2007, with the exception of two years during the mid-1990s and the five years following the Great Recession (Fuchs, 2012).

High levels of health care spending are problematic for the United States. Public spending on health care—primarily through the Medicare and Medicaid programs—is crowding out spending on other state and national priorities, including education, Social Security, national defense, and deficit reduction. Because health care represents such a large part of federal spending, it is considered a major driver of the budget deficit (Orszag, 2011). Health care spending also takes large bites out of state government budgets and substantially diminishes the discretionary spending of U.S. families (Auerbach and Kellermann, 2011).

High levels and high growth rates of U.S. health care spending have been attributed to numerous factors, including an aging population, increasing prevalence of chronic disease, and rising incomes. It has been estimated that increasing incomes and medical technology account for roughly one-quarter to one-half of spending growth since 1960 (Smith, Newhouse, and Freeland, 2009). Many health economists, including those at the Congressional Budget Office (CBO), cite growing use of advanced medical technologies as the most important driver of long-term growth in health care spending (CBO, 2008). As summarized in a recent review of the scholarly literature,

"The evidence suggests that over long periods of time a primary determinant of spending growth is the development, adoption and diffusion of new medical technology" (Chernew and Newhouse, 2012, p. 7).

In this report, we explore how new medical products affect spending in the United States and what this spending produces in terms of health improvement. We distinguish between "medical technology" and "medical products." We define *medical technology* broadly to include all applications of knowledge to practical medical problems. However, in this report we focus on *medical products*, which we define as drugs (including biologics, which include vaccines, blood products, or other therapies or diagnostic agents made from natural sources), devices (including diagnostics), and HIT.

From 2007 to 2011, the growth rate of U.S. spending on health care slowed to roughly the rate of inflation, leading some analysts and commentators to suggest that persistent spending growth rates exceeding GDP growth rates could be a thing of the past (Cutler and Sahni, 2013; Ryu et al., 2013). Moreover, data from CBO (2013, Table 2-1, p. 38) suggest that the annual growth rates of spending have declined over the past three decades. However, others maintain that optimism is premature, if not misplaced (Kaiser Family Foundation, 2013). As economist Victor Fuchs observes in a recent Perspective article in the *New England Journal of Medicine*, "every past prediction of a sustained slowing of the growth of health expenditures has been proved wrong" (Fuchs, 2012).

Whether the recent slowdown in health spending growth is temporary or will be more enduring is unknown. However, in either case, the fundamental premises of our study remain unaltered. Specifically, (1) some new medical products increase health care spending without also increasing health enough to warrant the extra spending, and (2) much of the utilization of some new products does not warrant the extra spending entailed. Considering the magnitude of annual U.S. health care spending and the consequences of those expenditures for other national priorities, it is well worth considering policy responses that could address these concerns.

As we argue in this report, the U.S. health care system provides strong incentives for U.S. medical product innovators to invent high-cost products and provides relatively weak incentives to invent low-cost ones. The resulting array of new medical products has profound implications not only for the United States and other high-income countries, but also for global health. This is because—with the exception of products to address medical conditions that are prevalent in low-income countries but not high-income ones—markets for drugs and devices in the United States and other high-income countries account for the lion's share of global sales and profits. As a result, profit-seeking innovators and their investors tend to focus their efforts on products that will generate profits in high-income countries. Changes in the U.S. health care system that offer greater financial rewards for inventing low-cost technologies—and less reward for inventing high-cost ones—could benefit patients across the globe.

Project Goals

Several previous reports (e.g., Schoen et al., 2007; Engelberg Center, 2013) have considered diverse policy options for limiting the growth of U.S. health care spending. We took a novel, and somewhat narrower, approach by focusing on what could be done to influence the mix of new medical products invented and offered for sale in the United States. Ongoing changes in factors that affect spending will change the growth rate of spending; in contrast, one-time changes will affect spending levels but not the spending growth rate (Chernew and Newhouse, 2012, pp. 5–6). Whether changes reduce the growth rate or the level of spending, the result is the same: Spending will be lower at any future time.

We had two policy goals:

1. Reduce total health care spending with the smallest possible loss of health benefits.
2. Ensure that new medical products that increase spending are accompanied by health benefits that are worth the spending increases.

Because the U.S. population is growing, progress toward the first goal will also reduce per capita spending. The second goal can be expressed in terms of achieving good value for any spending increases. These policy goals are distinct but related: Policy changes that affect how well we do with regard to one goal will often also affect how well we do with the other. (These social goals are distinct from economic efficiency, which we also accept as being important.)

To develop policy options for achieving the goals, we drew on a variety of information sources and methods:

- We reviewed scholarly and popular literature on medical product invention and utilization and used this information to characterize the context in which health care innovation occurs in the United States.
- We supplemented this information with data and insights from three additional sources:
  - interviews with health care industry leaders, product inventors, payers and insurers, investors, providers, and researchers
  - case studies of eight medical products
  - observations and advice from a technical expert panel (TEP) convened for this project.

We then synthesized this information to identify ten high-priority policy options that could encourage development of more products that would reduce health care spending, increase value, or accomplish both.

What Determines Value for Health Care Products?

The value of a new product depends on both its spending effects and the health effects from its actual use—in particular, the clinical circumstances under which it is used. For example, insulin offers high value only to people with diabetes. Antibiotics can be lifesaving when properly used to treat serious bacterial pneumonia, but they do nothing (and can even be harmful) if used to treat viral infections. Invasive diagnostic tests can detect disease at an early and treatable stage, but they can also cause serious complications or side effects. In sum, the value of a medical product depends on both its intrinsic properties and how appropriately it is used.

Depending on how well a new product performs and how well it is used, it may improve health and reduce aggregate or per capita health care spending. Such a product is desirable because it generates additional health for less money. But a new product could instead substantially increase spending while contributing little to improve health.

The principal tool for assessing the value of health care technologies is cost-effectiveness analysis (CEA; Gold et al., 1996; Sloan, 1996; A. Garber, 2000; Meltzer and Smith, 2012). CEA attempts to answer such questions as, "Between two alternative medical interventions that deliver the same kind of health improvements, which provides these benefits for a lower cost per unit of health improvement?" (A more technical discussion of CEA is included in Appendix A.) However, because our focus is health care spending, we adapted the methods of CEA to our goals. Under this interpretation, the price paid for a medical product affects its value; when other factors are equal, higher prices decrease value.

To make the concept of health improvements more concrete, we use the widely accepted construct of *quality-adjusted life years* (QALYs; Dolan, 2000). This yardstick seeks to quantify health effects in terms of extra years of life, adjusted to account for the quality of life during those years. The value of a health care product can then be expressed as the amount of additional spending required to achieve a given number of additional QALYs for the U.S. population, with both spending and health effects being expressed as differences in outcomes relative to the care that would have been delivered if the product were not used.

Reallocating resources to reduce health care spending or otherwise increase the value of new medical products may increase QALYs for many people, but others will be made worse off. For example, payers and/or providers could restrict use of a very expensive procedure using a particular medical device that has some positive benefit for some patients or a large benefit for a small number of patients. Many people would gain from such a change; others would lose. This fact makes pursuit of our policy goals controversial: Denying someone a costly but potentially health-improving treatment runs counter to the widely held belief that if patients want a treatment that might benefit them, they should be able to get it.

Many analysts have considered aggregate measures, such as national- or disease-level effects on health and costs or spending, to assess the value of medical technology in the United States (Cutler and McClellan, 2001; Cutler, 2004; Philipson et al., 2012). And they have typically concluded that additional costs or spending are justified by the associated health benefits, although the cost of an additional life year gained from medical care seems to have increased from the 1960s to the 1990s (Cutler, Rosen, and Vijan, 2006; A. Garber and Skinner, 2008).

Most important for our purposes, aggregate-level analyses can obscure important differences in the performance of different technologies used to fight particular diseases. Accordingly, our analyses focus on particular medical products. We explored how we can improve the mix of new products invented, encouraging those that are likely to decrease spending with only modest losses in health or that may generate substantial health benefits for modest spending increases.

Before we can explore ways to change the mix of medical products invented, we must understand the existing incentives and opportunities influencing the choices of medical product inventors and investors. In the next chapter, we begin to do so by describing the context for drug, device, and HIT innovation in the United States.

The Context for Medical Product Innovation

In this project, we considered U.S. spending and the health effects of medical products, whether invented in the United States or elsewhere. The medical products within the scope of our inquiry were new drugs (including biologics), devices (including diagnostics), and two kinds of HIT: EHRs and telemedicine. In this chapter we describe the context in which decisions about inventing such products are made, emphasizing the potential rewards that inventors can expect from selling their products and the influences of U.S. markets. We focus on U.S. markets because—unlike markets in other countries—the operation of these markets might be improved by policies under the control of U.S. policymakers.

This chapter contains more information about drugs and devices than about HIT. This is because there is active, ongoing discussion of policy options for improving HIT—especially EHRs—and policies to improve the effectiveness of EHRs in clinical decisionmaking are in flux (Executive Office of the President, 2010; FDA, 2013b; CMS, 2013c). Moreover, our telemedicine case study points to some well-known policy options for obtaining more value from telemedicine products. Because our research did not suggest policy options that would substantially augment the current policy discussion regarding HIT, we pay relatively little attention to HIT in this report.

Three Stages of Innovation

To identify ways to promote the invention of medical products that will be used in ways that decrease spending and are cost-effective, we need to understand the major forces that determine what medical products are invented and how they are used. In this chapter, we describe the key actors and influencers of product invention and use, what they do, and why.

We define medical product "innovation" as including the invention (or creation) of new products and making them available for use. We conceptualize the pathway to successful innovation as having three stages (Figure 2.1):

Figure 2.1
The Innovation Pathway

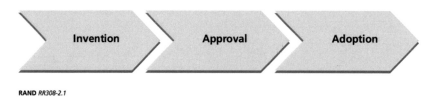

RAND *RR308-2.1*

1. creation of new products, which we call "invention"
2. regulatory approval for sale in the United States by the U.S. Food and Drug Administration (FDA)
3. processes that determine how and for which patients medical products are used, which we call "adoption" or "utilization."

Invention is strongly influenced by market forces, regulatory requirements, and other factors that determine the anticipated financial returns on investment for inventors and their private investors—and, thus, their financial incentives—as new products move through their life cycles. Collectively, these forces determine

- which new products are created, secure regulatory approval, and are adopted by health care providers
- the prices charged for new products
- the coverage, payment, and utilization management policies for new products, as determined by public and private payers
- which products are used for which patients
- how the new products affect health and spending.

In the following discussion, we highlight the decisions that seem most important in determining the targets of invention, FDA approval, adoption, health effects, spending, and ultimately the values of new medical products. We refer to the individuals and organizations that make the most important decisions as "primary actors" and those who seek to steer these decisions as "influencers." Primary actors at one stage of the innovation pathway may be influencers in another.

To understand the thinking of primary actors, we characterize their decisions in terms of goals and objectives, along with factors that either facilitate or constrain their actions.

Primary Actors in Inventing Medical Products

The primary actors in the invention of medical products include drug and device companies of various sizes and areas of focus, inventors of HIT, and private investors that provide financial resources to support invention.

Drug and Device Companies

Inventing new drugs involves two sets of activities. The first set, drug discovery, comprises efforts to identify promising molecules or "drug candidates" that display favorable biologic activity or are chemically similar to an effective agent. The second set of activities, drug development, involves a series of studies that determine whether a drug candidate demonstrates enough promise to be tested in humans—in the course of clinical trials—and subsequently demonstrates sufficient safety and efficacy to secure approval from the FDA for sale in the United States. In our terminology, drug discovery and drug development are two components of drug invention.

Pharmaceutical Companies

There are four major categories of drug companies:

- *"Big Pharma" companies* are multinational, and they invent drugs in several disease areas. Traditionally, these companies invented mostly small-molecule drugs that could be produced using chemical processes. Over the past decade or so, however, Big Pharma companies have greatly increased their efforts to invent biologic drugs (Tufts Center for the Study of Drug Development, 2013). They often buy the rights to drug candidates from other companies or enter into joint ventures with them to develop the candidates into commercial products. Big Pharma companies have the resources and expertise to shepherd promising drugs through the FDA review and approval processes and to market them.
- *Specialty companies* operate in one or a handful of disease areas or focus on categories of drugs with unusual characteristics. Many of these specialty drugs are biologics or "large-molecule" drugs that must be injected or infused—usually by a physician or other health care professional—rather than taken orally (Robinson, 2012).
- *Biotech companies* focus on drugs that are found in nature (large-molecule drugs), which tend to be considerably more costly to manufacture than small-molecule drugs. Where once these companies focused on refining naturally occurring molecules, such as human growth hormone, increasingly they rely on recombinant DNA and other production processes.
- *Start-up companies* are relatively small, fairly young firms that usually lack an FDA-approved product. These companies are often financed by individual investors, venture capital firms, or other private equity firms.

In 2012, global pharmaceutical sales, not factoring in discounts, totaled about $960 billion. Sales in the United States, Europe, and Japan accounted for about $325, $222, and $112 billion, respectively, which total about $659 billion—69 percent of global sales. Among the ten largest pharmaceutical companies in terms of U.S. sales in 2012, half are based in the United States, and half are based in Europe. The U.S. sales of those companies in 2012 ranged from about $12.5 to $20 billion. The therapeutic classes accounting for the largest U.S. sales include oncology drugs and mental health drugs, respiratory agents, antidiabetic drugs, and pain medications. (All figures are reported from tables downloaded from IMS Health [2014] or calculated by the authors from those data.)

Estimates of the average cost of discovering and developing a new drug vary widely—from roughly $150 million to $1.8 billion (Morgan et al. 2011). With costs of this size, private investors are unlikely to provide funds to invent a new drug unless they expect the effort to generate a healthy financial return, regardless of the drug's potential value to society.

Medical Device Companies

Medical devices include a wide array of products ranging from such everyday, low-risk products as bandages and wheelchairs to complex, expensive, and potentially high-risk diagnostic and therapeutic technologies, such as endoscopes and computed tomography (CT) scanners. Some devices are permanently implanted (e.g., pacemakers, stents, artificial joints), others are inserted for short periods of time (e.g., catheters, pumps, endoscopes), and still others are noninvasive (e.g., pulse oximeters, diagnostic imaging). Medical devices of primary interest in our analysis entail substantial levels of health care spending once they are adopted—primarily implanted devices and complex, expensive equipment.

At the beginning of the 21st century, the American medical-device industry—often referred to as "medtech"—comprised more than 6,000 companies and 3,000 product lines covering 50 clinical specialties. Many of these companies and product lines were very small. Only 64 product groups had revenues exceeding $150 million, and only 100 companies had annual revenues above $100 million. Seventy-two percent of medical device firms employed fewer than 50 people (Hanna, 2001). More recent industry statistics, attributed to Ernst & Young and reported by Makower, Meer, and Denend (2010), indicate that there are now roughly 1,000 medtech companies, with the leading product classes being cardiovascular and orthopedics.

Many device companies are founded by physician-entrepreneurs who receive early-stage funding from private investors. Entrepreneurs commonly enter the industry from academia or clinical practice or are former employees of large device manufacturers (Chatterji, 2008). Large device companies invent medical devices and acquire smaller medical device manufacturers whose technologies complement the bigger company's portfolio.

HIT Companies

HIT includes a wide range of products. They include those that create the information infrastructure for the U.S. health care system, as well as products for administrative (e.g., billing) purposes and products (such as decision support tools) that enable providers and patients to use that infrastructure in clinical care. To date, much of the activity in HIT has been in developing the infrastructure and administrative tools.

To effectively use the wide range of information relevant to clinical care, health data must be digitized, accessible, and transferable. Extensive adoption of EHRs would enable the development of other downstream HIT products and support a potential market for them. Several private companies invent EHRs. EHRs have also been created for internal use by such private and public health care providers as Kaiser Permanente and the U.S. Department of Veterans Affairs (VA).

Multiple EHR vendors offer products and services in the United States; for example, the Centers for Medicare & Medicaid Services (CMS) listed more than 20 vendors who are qualified to submit quality information to its Physician Quality Reporting System (CMS, 2013c). The Electronic Health Record Association, a trade group that represents companies that invent EHRs, has more than 40 member companies.

Much of the U.S. investment in inventing and adopting EHRs during the past few years has been spurred and shaped by money available from the federal government. More specifically, the Health Information Technology for Economic and Clinical Health (HITECH), part of the American Recovery and Reinvestment Act of 2009, provided $19 billion in incentives to spur adoption and "meaningful use" of EHRs. (See the electronic health records case study summary in Chapter Four.)

Goals of Medical Product Inventors

Inventors may be motivated by profits, altruism, academic advancement, prestige, or fame. But regardless of their fundamental motivations, inventors of products with substantial market potential in high-income countries generally want their products to be widely used in the United States. The U.S. market accounts for roughly one-third of global sales (derived from data reported in IMS Health, 2014). Since, on average, prices and profit margins on brand name drugs are almost certainly considerably higher in the United States than those in other countries, the U.S. market very likely contributes substantially more than one-third of global profits. Thus, prospects for U.S. adoption would be a major consideration for profit-seeking drug inventors and their private investors. (We have no analogous data for medical devices or HIT products.)

Private Investors

One important source of funding for invention is private investors in start-up drug and device companies. These investors usually provide cash in exchange for equity interests and management roles in start-up companies. Such investors include high net worth individuals, venture capital firms, other private equity firms, and pension and university investment funds. High net worth individuals invest their own money, while venture capital and private equity firms raise most of the money they invest from individual and institutional investors, such as pension funds. In order to be willing to invest, investors must anticipate an "attractive return on the capital invested" (Kocher and Roberts, 2014, p. 1).

Venture capitalists and other private equity companies typically seek to recoup their investments within roughly five years, through either a private sale of the company or through initial public offerings of stock. In general, venture capitalists are often said to target profit rates of 30 percent or more on their portfolio of investments (Robbins, Rudsenske, and Vaughan, 2008). Venture capitalists and corporate investors in medical devices typically seek annual returns of 40 percent or more (Zenios, Makower, and Yock, 2010, p. 684). Private investors seek—and often achieve—such high annual returns because of the degree of risk involved, including potential failure to create a commercially viable product, failure to secure regulatory approval in the United States, and long delays between investment and obtaining returns.

Ackerly et al. (2008) considered how public policies affect the ability of venture capital firms to raise funds to invest in health care companies. Almost all of their 20 fund-manager respondents reported that "the potential return given the risk" was either the only factor that mattered in their ability to raise funds, or that it mattered "very much" (p. w71). In addition, the authors reported that investors tend to prefer investing in devices rather than drugs or biotech because of "lower development costs, shorter development times, and reduced regulatory hurdles" (p. w71). Finally, the authors noted that "[r]espondents largely agreed on the importance of the relationship between returns and regulatory and reimbursement policies, ranking reimbursement, intellectual property protection, and the efficiency of the FDA review process as the most important risks affecting portfolio companies' returns" (p. w71). Notably, none of these considerations involves impacts on health that do not affect financial returns or effects on spending.

Some investors—such as public agencies and philanthropic foundations—are motivated by goals other than financial returns. For example, a public investment program may be focused on local economic development, and a foundation may be focused on improving health or reducing public spending. Nonetheless, we focus on private investors who are motivated by financial returns because changing their financial incentives appears to be a promising strategy by which to further our two policy goals.

Financial Incentives of Medical Product Inventors

It is the prospect of making profits that motivates companies to invest in product invention, and the more profit a company anticipates from a particular inventive effort, the greater is its incentive to commence or continue that effort. The profits a company can expect to earn from a particular product depend on the costs of inventing it (early in a product's life cycle), obtaining regulatory approval, and (later in the life cycle) revenues from selling the product anywhere in the world, net of its costs of production and marketing. Often when a company pursues a product-invention effort, it faces substantial uncertainty about invention costs, regulatory approval costs, the probability of bringing a product to market, and its net future revenue streams if it brings the product to market.

At each stage of the innovation pathway, new information becomes available that lessens or resolves some of this uncertainty. When new information arrives, the company may reassess whether to continue to invest in the product. A company may decide to cease an effort to invent and commercialize a new medical product for several reasons. First, the product invention effort may have encountered technical problems that render it impossible, excessively expensive, or too time consuming to create a commercially viable product. Second, after creating an apparently viable product, a company could decide not to pursue regulatory approval because the costs or time required to secure approval are too high. Finally, by the time a company receives regulatory approval, it may conclude that market conditions do not justify production and marketing costs—perhaps because a competitor has introduced a superior product. Companies will factor into their decisions the probabilities of a product failing at different points along the innovation pathway.

Companies decide whether to move forward at each stage of the innovation pathway based on their current assessments of the likelihoods of success, the market payoffs if they reach the adoption stage, and the additional cost of bringing the product to market. Expected future payoffs are adjusted to account for the costs of having money tied up and perhaps also to account for uncertainty. Thus, the financial incentive to embark on a product invention effort (1) is lower, other things being equal, when the expected costs of product invention, obtaining regulatory approval, and manufacturing and marketing the envisioned product are higher, and also when the anticipated amounts of time required for product invention and regulatory approval are higher; and (2) is higher, other things being equal, when the inventors are more confident that the product will get to market, generate higher annual net revenues, and generate revenues for a longer period of time. As we will see, because many products that could reduce spending have limited potential to generate profits, there appear to be inadequate incentives to invest in creating them. (A more technical discussion of decisionmaking by profit-seeking inventors is included in Appendix B.)

Influencers of Medical Product Invention

Multiple entities influence the decisions of inventors and investors in medical products.

National Institutes of Health

As the principal funder of basic biomedical research in the United States, the National Institutes of Health (NIH) invests substantial sums of money in extramural, investigator-initiated research that may provide insights leading to the discovery and development of drugs or invention of devices. Scientists employed by NIH and others funded by NIH also contribute more directly to drug development by discovering drug candidates. For example, in-house NIH researchers unlocked the secrets to developing an effective vaccine for *Haemophilus influenzae* type b (Hib; see the Hib case study summary in Chapter Four) and developed selective serotonin reuptake inhibitors, an important class of drugs for treating depression.

By virtue of its size and budget—approximately $31 billion per year—NIH is by far the largest federal investor in biomedical research. Other U.S. federal agencies play roles as well. These include the Centers for Disease Control, the U.S. Army Medical Research and Materiel Command, the Defense Advanced Research Projects Agency, the National Aeronautics and Space Administration, the Biomedical Advanced Research and Development Authority, and the National Science Foundation. Moreover, private U.S. companies and public and private organizations abroad conduct basic and applied research that facilitates efforts to invent new drugs and devices that may be adopted in the United States.

U.S. Food and Drug Administration

As the U.S. market gatekeeper for new prescription drugs and devices, as well as the regulator of labeling, manufacturing, and "indications" (i.e., the specific use[s] of a drug or device), the FDA exerts substantial influence on drug and device invention. Once a drug or device is approved for sale for a particular medical condition—the indication—doctors are free to use it "off label" for other purposes. Off-label use is very common. However, manufacturers face major restrictions on, and stiff penalties for, promoting products for off-label use (S. Garber, 2013, pp. 64–65). The FDA also grants periods of regulatory exclusivity that shield drug developers from competition, regardless of patents.

The FDA also regulates HIT products that are used in providing care. The agency is working with the Federal Communications Commission and the Office of the National Coordinator of Health Information Technology to develop "recommendations on an appropriate, risk-based regulatory framework for health IT [information technology] that promotes innovation, protects patient safety, and avoids unnecessary and duplicative regulations" (FDA, 2013b). As part of this effort (as of February 2014), the agency was also developing draft guidance for manufacturers on interoperability of medical devices (Lee, 2014).

U.S. Patent and Trademark Office

Patents can be critical facilitators of new drug and device invention (Graham et al., 2009; Zenios, Makower, and Yock, 2010, pp. 210–272; Goldman and Lakdawalla, 2012). The U.S. Patent and Trademark Office (USPTO) is responsible for reviewing and granting applications for U.S. patents. Patent holders have a legal right of up to 20 years from the time of application filing to exclude others from using the subject matter covered by their patents. However, this right can be very costly to enforce because it can require pursuing lawsuits in the federal courts. Thus, patents are an imperfect, albeit often effective, means of protecting new drugs and devices from competition.

The policy motivation for providing patent protection is to encourage investment in inventions by reducing the risk that profits will be eroded early in a product's life cycle by competition from imitators. However, a patent can be a double-edged sword. In the context of pharmaceuticals, patents on research tools that drug developers want to use can substantially increase invention costs. In addition, device inventors are frequently targeted by patent holders claiming infringement of their patents.

Office of the National Coordinator for Health Information Technology

Located within the Office of the Secretary for the U.S. Department of Health and Human Services (HHS), the Office of the National Coordinator for Health Information Technology (ONC) is responsible for promoting the use of HIT and electronic exchange of health information. Key responsibilities of ONC are the development of meaningful use (MU) standards for EHRs and the administration of HIT adoption programs. ONC directly influences the invention of HIT by providing funding to inventors. In addition, ONC has awarded prizes to inventors who were able to meet particular HIT challenges. Moreover, the rules for MU are used to determine which providers are eligible for payments to subsidize their EHR adoptions. The availability of such payments tends to substantially increase demand for systems that meet the MU standards, and, as a result, EHR designs are likely to be substantially influenced by those standards.

Primary Actor and Influencers in Approval of Medical Technologies

The primary actor at the approval stage is the FDA, which ultimately decides what products will reach the U.S. market and with what approved indications. The stakes to manufacturers in FDA actions are very high, including whether their products will be approved at all and, if so, how much time and money the approval will require. A drug or device manufacturer interacts with the FDA throughout the product invention and regulatory review process. Such interactions are likely to affect the duration and, less often, the outcome of a particular review. Moreover, drug and device companies try to influence FDA policy broadly through such channels as public affairs activities, lobbying, and congressional testimony. In addition, politicians often try to influence the FDA through public criticism of its decisions, especially when an approved drug or device turns out to cause large numbers of severe injuries.

Primary Actors in Adoption of Medical Products

The financial and other rewards that flow to inventors and investors are determined by what happens to new medical technologies in the market once they are available for sale. Whether inventors have positive impacts on society, while also achieving substantial returns on their time and money investments, depends in large measure on whether and how widely products are adopted and used by health care providers, such as physicians and hospitals.

Physicians

Physicians pursue personal financial rewards in tandem with wanting to do what is best for their patients (Chandra and Skinner, 2012). These financial rewards have major effects on utilization of health care products. For example, fee-for-service (FFS) payment approaches—which are still widely used by Medicare and many private insurers—in effect reward physicians who provide more services, whether or not they are truly beneficial. When payment amounts are generous, physicians have a powerful incentive to provide treatments that are beneficial to some individuals and also to others who are unlikely to benefit much, if at all. (This is an aspect of a phenomenon called "treatment creep" that is discussed in Chapter Four.)

Physicians also decide whether to adopt EHR systems and telemedicine products for use in their offices. They may also advise the hospitals in which they practice about the advantages and disadvantages of EHR and telemedicine systems.

Specialty pharmaceuticals (e.g., chemotherapy drugs) provide examples of how payment policies, coupled with physician desire for income, can increase spending. Specialty pharmaceuticals are usually large-molecule drugs that are administered (injected or infused) to patients by physicians. Policies governing their use provide substantial incentives for physician practices to administer these agents (Robinson, 2012). For example, in addition to providing a procedure-based payment for intravenously administering such drugs, Medicare pays medical oncologists 106 percent of the average price paid for the chemotherapy drugs they use. This arrangement rewards physicians for using the most expensive drug in any class of chemotherapy agents (see the case study summary in Chapter Four on the use of Avastin to treat breast cancer; Scott Morton and Kyle, 2012, p. 813).

Hospitals

To distribute their high overhead costs, hospitals have strong incentives to fill every bed, and with well-insured patients especially. To fill beds, hospital administrators need community physicians to admit patients to their facilities, rather than those of competitors. One well-known and expensive ramification of this dynamic is the "medical arms race." The term refers to the tendency of many hospitals (and other health care facilities) to compete for community physicians and their patients by acquiring the latest, high-tech—and often expensive—diagnostic and therapeutic technologies. (See the case study summary on robotic surgery in Chapter Four.)

To the extent that factors other than community doctor preferences determine which hospital gets patients, the arms race slows. For example, in the 1990s, insurance companies successfully bargained with hospitals by threatening not to cover admissions of their enrollees and forced hospitals that wanted to be in the insurers' network to accept lower payments (Keeler, Melnick, and Zwanziger, 1999). Later, hospital chains in many health care markets used their size and increased bargaining power to break the insurance companies' grip on payments (Melnick and Keeler, 2007).

Two developments that could slow the medical arms race are hospital acquisition of physician practices and the creation of accountable care organizations (ACOs)—integrated delivery systems created to compete for Medicare beneficiaries and newly insured patients covered through the health exchanges established by the Affordable Care Act (ACA).

Individual incentives matter too. Consider payments to hospital CEOs. Specifically, "Across the nation, boards at nonprofit hospitals . . . are often paying bosses much more for boosting volume than for delivering value" (Hancock, 2013). To counter the tendency to provide unnecessary tests and procedures, CMS and many other payers give hospital facilities a fixed "prospective payment" for an admission in each of the hundreds of diagnostic related groups (DRGs), based on the national average cost for that group. In 2000, Medicare adopted a prospective payment system for care delivered by hospitals on an outpatient basis (CMS, 2012). Prospective payment gives hospitals strong incentives to hold down costs for each admission—and thereby increases demand for some low-cost medical products—for example, by avoiding purchases of high-cost equipment and unnecessary treatments, as well as reducing average lengths of stay. However, prospective payment is not a panacea because, for example, it does not restrain numbers of hospital admissions or which patients are treated.

Hospitals decide which EHR systems to adopt or create in house and which telemedicine products to purchase. They also decide which administrative (e.g., billing) and clinical decision-support capabilities they want to incorporate in their EHR systems.

Influencers of Providers

Product inventors, such as drug and device manufacturers and EHR vendors, seek to influence physicians by collaborating with physician thought leaders (Spurling et al., 2010) and by direct marketing aimed at both prescribers and patients. Research indicates that marketing to physicians affects prescribing behavior (Spurling et al., 2010).

Patients sometimes try to influence physician decisions regarding their care. On average, those with more generous insurance receive more care than less generously insured patients (Newhouse and the Insurance Experiment Group, 1993). Also, there is evidence that drug and device marketing to consumers—called direct-to-consumer advertising—increases utilization (Scott Morton and Kyle, 2012, p. 818).

Still, many providers appear not to take patient preferences into account. For example, most patients prefer to receive less aggressive care than most physicians prefer to provide (Chandra, Cutler, and Song, 2012, p. 411). However, many patients tend to associate more care, higher cost, and newer technology with higher quality (Korobkin, 2012, p. 25).

Public and private payers also influence providers' utilization decisions. These payers include insurers and self-insured organizations—such as employers and unions—that bear the financial risk for groups of people. Payers decide for their populations (1) what technologies and services are *eligible for payment* (that is, "covered" but not necessarily fully reimbursed), which for private payers often depends on how they interpret and apply such contractual terms as "medically necessary," (2) the clinical circumstances or *patient selection criteria* under which a particular technology is covered, and (3) the *utilization management* policies and processes used to enforce their coverage rules.

CMS, which administers Medicare and Medicaid, is the largest single payer in the United States. Medicare and Medicaid account for almost one-third of all U.S. health care spending. Under the statutory language governing Medicare, medical technologies and associated services are covered (for particular patients) if they are "reasonable and necessary for the diagnosis or treatment of illness or injury or to improve the functioning of a malformed body member" (Neumann et al., 2005, p. 244). Medicare is not allowed to consider costs in making coverage decisions (Neumann and Chambers, 2012).

For some devices and associated procedures, particularly those "deemed particularly controversial or projected to have a major impact on the program" (Neumann et al., 2005, p. 244), CMS makes "national coverage determinations" (Neumann et al., 2005; Zenios, Makower, and Yock, 2010, p. 511). These determinations, once made, make it difficult for Medicare to reverse its coverage decisions—even if subsequent evidence suggests that the harms from a technology's use outweigh its potential benefits. (See the case study summary on prostate-specific antigen [PSA] screening in Chapter Four.) For the large majority of technologies for which no national coverage determination is made, Medicare contractors make local coverage determinations guided by the broad statutory criteria (Foote, 2003; Neumann et al., 2005; Neumann and Chambers, 2012).

Medicare policies influence coverage decisions of many private payers. More specifically, in many instances private payers follow Medicare's lead (S. Garber et al., 2000; Zenios, Makower, and Yock, 2010, p. 513) in deciding whether to cover a technology. As a result, changes in Medicare policy can affect health and spending for patients who are not insured by Medicare.

Private payers, including those offering Medicare (Part C) Advantage plans, substantially influence use of medical products. Private payers typically delegate drug coverage decisions to pharmacy and therapeutics committees or to pharmacy benefit management companies (PBMs). Covered drugs are usually listed in a formulary along with the clinical circumstances under which drugs are covered. Private payers use direct and indirect methods to keep drug utilization in line with their coverage policies. Direct methods include prior authorization and step therapy (i.e., less expensive drugs must be tried unsuccessfully before more expensive ones may be used). Indirect methods include patient cost-sharing, which affects patients' decisions about use of both necessary and unnecessary care (Chandra, Cutler, and Song, 2012, p. 408), and drug utilization review (administrative checks on which patients get which drugs).

Different payment structures or approaches confront providers with different incentives that affect their utilization of medical products. For example, Medicare Advantage plans and health systems that provide both insurance and medical services are "capitated"—i.e., they accept a fixed payment per enrollee for which they agree to provide all needed care, subject to modest cost-sharing and restrictions. Such organizations have an incentive to reduce the costs of care, while also providing quality care to encourage current members to stay and new members to join. The tension between the objectives of pleasing members and lowering costs makes it worthwhile for these organizations to avoid low-value services.

Payers have used other financial arrangements to encourage providers to reduce costs and/or raise quality. For example, some insurers pay more for better performance, as measured by both cost and quality criteria. Similarly, CMS is experimenting with ACOs, which take some responsibility for FFS Medicare patients and share savings if they can keep actual costs below expected costs. The VA and its component facilities have similar incentives insofar as they are given payments in advance, in return for which they are supposed to provide care for a defined population as efficiently as possible.

Office of the National Coordinator for Health Information Technology: Hospitals and physician offices are eligible for incentive payments for adoption of EHRs that conform to ONC's EHR meaningful use standards. Medical professionals can receive up to $44,000 over five years under the Medicare incentive program or up to $63,750 over six years under the Medicaid program. The availability of these incentives has almost certainly increased EHR adoption. HHS reported that as of April 2013, nearly 80 percent of eligible hospitals and over half of eligible providers had received an incentive payment (HHS, 2013).

Summary: Context for Medical Product Innovation

Figure 2.2 provides an overview of the discussion in this chapter. The figure overlays the innovation pathway in Figure 2.1 with examples of the key decisionmakers and influencers at each stage. As suggested by the feedback arrow, the incentives of inventors and investors are shaped by what they anticipate about the adoption and utilization of their potential inventions, which determine the expected market rewards for those inventions and the risks associated with those rewards.

In sum, the financial incentives of inventors and investors as they decide which new products to try to invent depend critically on the intrinsic qualities of the invention, as well as how it is used. How quickly an innovation is adopted and how it is used are determined by providers, whose behavior is shaped in turn by their own financial incentives and by manufacturers, patients, and payers. Expectations about approval and adoption of a technology shape the decisions of innovators and investors. This basic framework provides the foundation for our analysis.

The next chapter describes our analytic approach and key information sources.

Figure 2.2
Key Actors and Influencers Along the Innovation Pathway

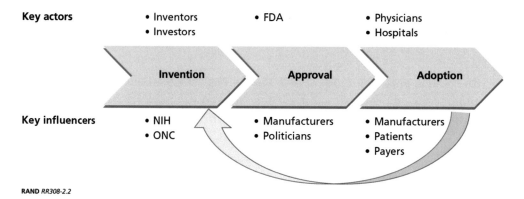

CHAPTER THREE

Methods

Using a variety of methods, we explored how new medical products affect U.S. health care spending and relationships between spending changes caused by the availability of medical products and the associated changes in U.S. population health. Then we sought to identify policy options that could improve the existing mix of incentives for product invention.

We conducted literature reviews to identify key issues in product invention, understand the context for medical product invention, and generate a preliminary list of policy options. We supplemented this information with 50 one-on-one interviews with health care industry leaders, drug and device inventors, regulators, health care payers and insurers, venture capitalists, and researchers. To illustrate how various forces influence the invention and use of medical products, we also conducted case studies of eight health care products. The case studies highlight how products can succeed or fail in the health care marketplace.

Literature Reviews

At the outset of the project, we reviewed a wide and diverse body of peer-reviewed and other literature on the invention and adoption of medical products. From this review, we synthesized an understanding of the drivers of medical product invention and adoption in the United States; products' effects on spending; and public and private policies that impede, enable, or reward invention of products with different effects on value.

To illustrate how these forces play out, we developed a framework for describing the environment in which innovation takes place in the United States. We paid special attention to how new policies and incentives, or modification of existing ones, might encourage inventors to focus on creating medical products that could reduce spending with little sacrifice in health or otherwise generate good value when commercialized in the United States. We considered issues related to adoption of medical products insofar as these can, in the short term, (1) deliver substantial improvements in value over existing technologies and (2) reward inventors for creating products that could help reduce health care spending in the medium to long term.

Technical Expert Panel

To help us achieve our project goals, we convened a panel of national experts to review our ideas and weigh the promise of various policy options suggested by our findings. The panel included leaders from the fields of medical technology development; private financing; the adoption, diffusion, and assessment of health care technologies; health system administration; and public policy. Two panel meetings were held. The first, which took place in Santa Monica, California, in January 2013, focused on the study's goals, aims, methods, and analytical plan. The panel offered comments on our draft analytical framework, weighed the pros and cons of different case study topics, and suggested several policy options. The second meeting, held in Seattle, Washington, in November 2013, focused on reviewing and discussing the team's findings and discussing a list of potential policy options.

Members of the Technical Expert Panel

Donald M. Berwick, M.D.	President Emeritus and Senior Fellow, Institute for Healthcare Improvement, Cambridge, Massachusetts
Otis W. Brawley, M.D., F.A.C.P.	Emory University and American Cancer Society
Philippe Chambon, M.D., Ph.D.	Managing Director, New Leaf Venture Partners LLC
Delos M. Cosgrove, M.D.	CEO and President, Cleveland Clinic
Ezekiel J. Emanuel, M.D., Ph.D.	Vice Provost for Global Initiatives; Diane v.S. Levy and Robert M. Levy University Professor; Chair, Department of Medical Ethics and Health Policy, University of Pennsylvania
Atul Gawande, M.D., M.P.H.	Surgeon, Brigham and Women's Hospital; Director, Ariadne Labs; Professor, Harvard School of Public Health and Harvard Medical School
Brent C. James, M.D., M.Stat.	Chief Quality Officer, Intermountain Healthcare
Dean Kamen	Founder and President of DEKA Research & Development Corporation

Karen Katen	Senior Advisor, Essex Woodlands
Larry Kessler, Sc.D.	Professor and Chair, Department of Health Services, School of Public Health, University of Washington
Vinod Khosla	Partner, Khosla Ventures
Kenneth W. Kizer, M.D., M.P.H.	Distinguished Professor, University of California (UC) Davis School of Medicine and Betty Irene Moore School of Nursing; Director, Institute for Population Health Improvement, UC Davis Health System
Robert Langer	Massachusetts Institute of Technology
Mark McClellan, M.D., Ph.D.	Senior Fellow and Director, Initiative on Value and Innovation in Health Care, The Brookings Institution
Arnold Milstein, M.D.	Professor of Medicine, Clinical Excellence Research Center Director, Stanford University
Trevor Mundel, M.D., Ph.D.	President, Global Health, Bill & Melinda Gates Foundation
Peter J. Neumann, Sc.D.	Director, Center for the Evaluation of Value and Risk in Health, Institute for Clinical Research and Health Policy Studies, Tufts Medical Center; Professor, Tufts University School of Medicine
Boris Nikolic, M.D.	Chief Advisor for Science and Technology to Bill Gates
Michael A. Peterson	President and Chief Operating Officer, Peter G. Peterson Foundation
Michael E. Porter	Professor, Harvard Business School

Expert Interviews

To add depth to our analysis; explore concepts drawn from published literature about the realities of product invention, investing, and U.S. health care markets; and understand the latest developments and trends, we conducted 50 in-depth interviews with health care industry experts, drug and device inventors, regulators, payers and insurers, venture capitalists, and researchers, many of whom are listed (with their permission) in the Acknowledgments of this report. These interviews, which drew upon each expert's firsthand knowledge, had two major aims:

1.   to gather detailed information on the determinants of medical product invention and adoption
2.   to identify and explore existing and potential political, institutional, and market enablers and barriers to inventing products that could reduce spending or otherwise provide high value.

Between May and October 2013, we conducted 30- to 60-minute semistructured interviews with each expert, using protocols tailored for each of seven areas. The protocols are available as an online appendix at www.rand.org/t/RR308. Each protocol addressed issues related to the invention and use of medical products, but the focus differed depending on the expert's background. We interviewed

- high-level general policy experts, including government officials (13)
- device inventors (6)
- drug inventors (6)
- HIT inventors (4)
- investors in new medical products (7)
- payment and coverage experts (7)
- providers (7).

Interviewees included representatives from pharmaceutical and medical device research and marketing units; current and past FDA officials; and heads of smaller entrepreneurial enterprises, venture capital firms, and start-ups. A note-taker was present for all interviews. While we endeavored to interview experts with widely ranging perspectives and opinions, our samples of interview subjects are not representative of all potential subjects within a category.

Our 50 interviewees were determined as follows. First, we created the categories (listed in the previous paragraph) of topics or areas of expertise about which we wanted to learn more. Within each category (e.g., drug invention), we sought a range of perspectives. Then we brainstormed to identify well-regarded people with extensive expertise in each category whom we anticipated would have diverse experiences and perspectives. We invited 72 experts to participate in interviews; five explicitly declined, and 17 others did not respond. In a few cases, we did not follow up with nonresponders because we had already conducted enough interviews in the relevant category; in the other cases, we were unable to schedule interviews.

The interview notes were reviewed and considered along with information from the case studies and literature to develop our study themes, which are discussed in Chapter Four. The interview notes were then coded and analyzed according to the themes. Because interviewees were assured that we would not quote them by name, throughout the report we paraphrase their comments, indicated by italics, and reference them only by a code reflecting the interview category combined with a unique number for each interviewee in that category (e.g., GENX1). The codes are defined as follows:

- GENX: general health care policy expert
- DEV: device inventor
- DRUG: drug inventor
- HIT: health information technology inventor
- INVES: private investor
- COV: coverage expert
- PROV: provider.

In some cases, we report the views of particular interview subjects even if they seem to conflict with more reliable information, such as peer-reviewed studies. Nonetheless, in conducting our analyses, we remained cognizant of the possibility that interviewees sometimes lacked objectivity because they did not take account of issues that were not important to them or because they and their organizations had private stakes in public policies that could upset a status quo under which they were doing well.

Case Studies

To help illustrate our analytical framework and more specific issues, we selected eight products that provide examples of how different steps in the innovation pathway influence the invention, approval, and adoption of new medical products, as well as their ultimate impacts on U.S. spending and health.

We compiled an extensive list of case study candidates. In developing this list, we sought to encompass variation across case studies regarding several criteria. These criteria included the disease(s) involved, barriers to innovation, the timing and extent of U.S. adoption, and the impacts on health and health care spending in the United States.

We then discussed the candidates with our technical expert panel at their first meeting. Based on their feedback and further discussion, we selected eight inventions: three drugs (including one biologic), three devices (a diagnostic, an implantable, and a costly machine), and two health information technologies:

- Avastin for metastatic breast cancer
- a cardiovascular polypill
- electronic health records
- the *Haemophilus influenzae* type b (Hib) vaccine
- implantable cardioverter-defibrillators (ICDs)
- prostate-specific antigen
- robotic surgery
- telemedicine.

These products are not a random sample from a population of medical products, nor are they representative of potential new drugs, devices, or HIT products. For these reasons, we use the case studies for illustration, not inference.

The detailed case studies are available as online appendixes at www.rand.org/t/ RR308. Short summaries of the case studies are interspersed in Chapters Four and Five.

To undertake each case study, we commissioned physician authors with a relevant specialty background and additional training in health services research. All of the authors were either research fellows or recent graduates of the Robert Wood Johnson Clinical Scholars program. Authors were asked to use a standard framework that addressed each of the following dimensions:

- Definition: a definition or description of the product
- Rationale: What need was the product devised to address?
- Genesis: early development, including how the work was funded
- Early adoption: Who adopted the product, and what regulatory hurdles were involved?
- Dissemination: How quickly did the use of the product spread? What factors (intrinsic to the technology or extrinsically applied) promoted or restricted its uptake and use?
- Impact: What is known about the product's impact on health outcomes, complications, and costs?

In the course of compiling their case studies, the authors interacted with a supervising editor (Arthur Kellermann). National or international experts with special knowledge of the topic were asked to review particular case studies to identify any errors of omission or commission.

Policy Options

In Chapter Four, we use information from the literature, interviews, and technical expert panel members to develop five themes highlighting features of the U.S. health care environment that affect the incentives of primary actors. To develop the policy options presented in Chapter Five, we considered policy options suggested in the literature, by technical expert panel members, and by interviewees and then identified and analyzed problems encompassed by the themes that might be mitigated through changes in public and private policy to advance our two policy goals.

CHAPTER FOUR

Analysis

The decisions made by inventors of and investors in new medical products are driven by two key considerations. The first is a technical assessment of whether the new technology can be successfully brought to market. The probability of success is influenced by perceptions of two types of risks: scientific risk (Will the technology work?) and regulatory risk (Will the government approve it for use?).

The second consideration is financial: Are the expected payoffs large enough to justify the costs incurred to bring the product to market? As we suggested in Chapter Two, the answer to this question is greatly influenced by the decisions of medical providers, who are, in turn, influenced by their own financial considerations. This view is supported by research and popular literature, as well as by our interviews, case studies, and much of the discussion at the two meetings of the technical expert panel. Thus, our strategy for increasing value is to identify policies, described in Chapter Five, that could alter the expected costs and rewards, as well as the technical, regulatory, and market risks perceived by the key actors who determine which products are invented.

To promote understanding of these issues, we distilled five themes from the information we collected and synthesized:

- lack of basic scientific knowledge
- costs and risks of FDA approval
- inadequate rewards for medical products that could decrease spending
- treatment creep
- the medical arms race.

The themes refer to features of the U.S. health care environment that substantially affect the costs and risks of, and rewards for, medical product invention. We explain how these costs and rewards influence the degree to which U.S. health care spending increases current and future population health.

The first two themes relate to whether a product can be successfully brought to market and the costs and risks of doing so. The last three describe aspects of U.S. markets for medical products and health care that either (1) limit the market rewards that inventors and investors expect for inventing products that decrease spending or otherwise provide high value or (2) provide large market rewards for low-value products.

We now consider each theme, integrating related information from the interviews and using information from case studies to illustrate and elaborate.

Lack of Basic Scientific Knowledge

We define *basic science* as systematic investigations aimed at increasing knowledge that do not involve any specific, practical goals. Some fields of basic sciences that can lead to knowledge applicable to the invention of medical products include anatomy, physiology, genetics, pathology, virology, biochemistry, materials science, solid and fluid mechanics, software engineering, and electronics. To successfully invent new medical products, inventors rely upon and apply basic scientific knowledge. Recent empirical studies provide evidence that basic and clinical research funded by NIH stimulates product development efforts by pharmaceutical companies (Toole, 2007; Blume-Kohout, 2012). Invention of medical devices also requires substantial knowledge of the disease that the device would ameliorate (Zenios, Makower, and Yock, 2010, pp. 61, 145).

In many instances, scientific understanding of the biological processes underlying diseases is not sufficient to support investments in product invention. This is because lack of sufficient knowledge greatly increases the likely costs of invention, the time required to invent, and the likelihood of failing to find an effective solution.

One interviewee [DRUG2] with a background in drug development and investment noted that *academic and small-company innovators are driven secondarily by profit [and] market size—issues that have a higher priority in a big company. These are innovators who are driven by underlying scientific questions.* Nonetheless, while many academics and early-stage medical product inventors are motivated by a desire to "do good" or a passion for science, financial resources are usually needed to support inventive efforts when push comes to shove, as some of our interviews emphasized.

Many of our interviewees emphasized that *investors, as well as drug and device developers, assess the "probability of technical success"* [INVES6] regularly in deciding whether to invest or continue investing. The risk assessments done at the early stages are critical because, as one interviewee put it, *an early "no" saves a company a lot more money than a later "no"* [DRUG1].

Lack of an Adequate Knowledge Base Can Hinder Product Inventors

Given the calculus of investment decisions, medical product invention for a disease is unlikely to progress until there is a solid base of scientific knowledge related to the underlying disease processes. In principle, new scientific knowledge in the public domain could be the springboard that triggers efforts to apply this knowledge to the invention of new medical products.

Sources of Financial Support for Increasing Basic Scientific Knowledge

Basic biomedical knowledge is developed by businesses hoping to apply that knowledge to invent new products, by academic scientists, and by collaborations or partnerships between them. Much of the literature suggests that drug and device companies conduct little basic science, largely limiting their activities to applying basic scientific knowledge created by others, especially academic research labs. Such labs receive financial support from many sources, including NIH, other federal research agencies, drug and device companies, and philanthropists.

However, some of our interviews indicated that some drug and device companies do conduct basic scientific research. For example, an interview subject [DRUG1] with extensive experience in Big Pharma reported that *drug companies spend more of their R&D [research and development] budgets on basic science than most people think, particularly in discovering (as contrasted with developing) potential drugs, much of which involves identifying drug targets (such as various kinds of enzymes) or biological processes that a drug might alter to achieve a desirable effect on a patient.* This view was echoed by another of our experts [DRUG6]. According to one interviewee [DEV6], in the device world *early-stage venture capital investments are considered extensions of the R&D pipeline, supporting early research and development activities.* That interviewee also expressed concern that venture capitalists have *recently pulled back early-stage device investing and that R&D activity has been curtailed as a result* (an issue also mentioned by DEV5).

Federal Funding Is Critical to Expanding the Basic Scientific Base

NIH is the world's leading source of funding for biomedical research. Most NIH funding is provided (as "extramural" grants) to non-NIH investigators, who work primarily at U.S. academic institutions. In 2011, NIH spent about seven times as much on extramural research grants as on intramural research (NIH, Office of Budget, 2013).

However, the Hib case study on the following page illustrates the potential value of intramural NIH research activity, which provided the scientific breakthrough underpinning the development of Hib conjugate vaccines. This case study also illustrates the potential value of partnerships between government agencies and private industry, which in this instance resulted in an innovation that produced enormous health benefits per dollar spent. (We have no information about payoffs to NIH intramural research more broadly.)

Haemophilus influenzae Type b (Hib) Vaccine

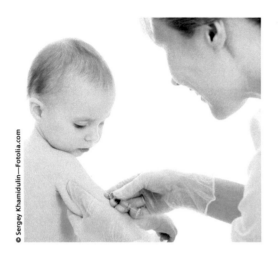

© Sergey Khamidulin—Fotolia.com

The Technology: *Haemophilus influenzae* type b (Hib) infection was a major cause of death and disability among infants and young children in the United States and worldwide. It was the leading cause of acquired intellectual disability. With the best available treatment, it caused death in about 10 percent of patients in the United States; 30 percent of the recovered had permanent neurological and behavioral outcomes. Development of Hib vaccines transformed this picture. Today, fewer than 100 cases of Hib infection occur each year in the United States. The vaccine is composed of the capsular polysaccharide (outer layer) of the Hib bacterium chemically bound to a carrier protein. Injected, it elicits a protective immune response, even in infants with immature immune systems. Protection is lifelong.

Infants and Young Children Are the Most Vulnerable: In the United States, prior to the use of the Hib vaccine, unvaccinated 6- to 12-month-old infants sustained the highest rates of Hib disease, when maternally transferred antibodies waned and the self-generated antibodies had not yet evolved. The first generation of Hib polysaccharide-only vaccine provoked a protective immune response in older children and adults; however, it failed to stimulate enough antibodies in children younger than 18 months. The FDA and the Centers for Disease Control and Prevention (CDC) endorsed the vaccine's use. More than 10 million doses of the Hib polysaccharide vaccine were administered in the United States between 1985 and 1989 (Peltola, 2000), when they were supplanted by newer, more effective second-generation vaccines.

Second-Generation Vaccines Represent a Major Breakthrough: When researchers linked the Hib capsular polysaccharide to a carrier protein, the resulting "conjugate" vaccine evoked a powerful immune response, even in infants. The first conjugate Hib vaccine was licensed in 1987 and swiftly supplanted the first-generation vaccines. Multiple studies documented high rates of protection against Hib disease, at all age groups. Research done in both developed and developing countries showed that Hib conjugate vaccines are highly effective at preventing Hib infection and even nasopharyngeal carriage, an important way that the disease is passed from one child to another.

Cost-Benefit Trade-Off: In the developed world, the benefits of the vaccine clearly surpass its costs. By 2002, Hib conjugate vaccines had reduced the burden of Hib disease by 99 percent in the United States. Similar benefits have been noted in other Western countries that achieved high rates of vaccination. In developing countries, the vaccine usage is partial and increasing slowly; as a result, Hib disease continues to kill an estimated 600,000 infants every year.

A Technology "Home Run": The CDC designated vaccines universally recommended for children as one of the country's ten great public health achievements of the 20th century (Centers for Disease Control and Prevention, 1999b). Hib vaccine leads the list (Centers for Disease Control and Prevention, 1999a). The Hib vaccine has saved the lives of tens of thousands of American children, reduced the incidence of catastrophic complications, and virtually eliminated what was once the leading cause of acquired intellectual disability in the United States. If a comprehensive vaccination program could be mounted, it might be possible to eradicate Hib infection worldwide.

The Eunice Kennedy Shriver National Institute of Child Health and Human Development (NICHD) considers development of the Hib vaccine one of its greatest contributions to public health. Hib conjugate vaccines broadly exemplify the value of partnerships between public research agencies (in this case, the intramural and extramural research programs of NICHD and the National Institute of Allergy and Infectious Diseases), public health (the CDC, which conducted important epidemiological and efficacy studies), the FDA (which reviewed and approved the marketing of the first- and second-generation polysaccharide vaccines), and private industry (which provided the technical sophistication to develop additional protein conjugates, the resources to test them, and the production and marketing capacity to widely disseminate Hib conjugate vaccines throughout the United States, the developed world, and, perhaps in time, worldwide).

How Scientific Uncertainty Affects Medical Product Invention

It seems that many high-burden diseases lack effective treatment primarily because scientific understanding of disease processes falls short of what product inventors think is required to justify large-scale investments. As described by one interviewee [DRUG4], *when making decisions about where to invest research and development resources, developers consider "Where is the science currently? Is that an achievable intervention?" Take the extreme example of Alzheimer's—we thought we understood more than we actually do. The bar has gotten quite high.*

This is not to deny that the potential market reward is also a key component of incentives to invent. For example, despite the fact that the biology of Alzheimer's disease is poorly understood, several companies are trying to develop drugs for this disease (PhRMA, 2013; Coombs, 2013), and the FDA is considering how to ease rules for approval of Alzheimer's drugs (Kozauer and Katz, 2013; Kolata, 2013). Thus, policy options for expanding basic biomedical knowledge are worth exploring.

Costs and Risks of FDA Approval

Under U.S. law, inventors of prescription drugs, medical devices, and some HIT products must gain approval from the FDA before offering their products for sale in the United States. Approval is based on processes that the FDA views as necessary to guarantee product safety and efficacy. Almost all stakeholders agree that regulation to ensure safety is essential; there is less agreement about ensuring efficacy. However, there is controversy about whether the FDA could ensure the safety of medical products while reducing the direct costs and delays necessitated by the product review and approval processes. The FDA deserves credit for doing a really difficult job well. Because our interest centers on how to improve FDA regulation to further our policy goals, our discussion focuses on potential problems that might be addressed to further these goals.

Industry groups, drug and device companies, inventors, and investors have expressed two major concerns: (1) the time and monetary costs of obtaining FDA approval and (2) the unpredictability of FDA requirements for approvals in specific cases.

Could the FDA Ensure Safety with Quicker and Less Costly Processes?

A long-standing and controversial claim is that the FDA review and approval processes take considerably longer and require more information from manufacturers than is necessary to ensure that products are sufficiently safe and efficacious to be sold in the United States. The substantial financial and time costs associated with satisfying the FDA regulatory process stem primarily from the extent and nature of the information that the inventor must develop and provide to the FDA to support safety and efficacy review and the time the FDA needs to conduct careful and thorough reviews.

Delays Entail Both Health and Financial Costs

During the time before a medical product is available for sale, its health benefits are denied to patients for whom the product would be the best diagnostic, treatment, or preventive option (Peltzman, 1974; Grabowski and Vernon, 1983; Calfee et al., 2008; Philipson and Sun, 2008). Until the FDA approves a product for U.S. marketing, financial returns, if any, on the capital invested in product invention must come from foreign markets.

Several interviewees opined that the amount of evidence required from applicants is greater for some products than for others. One interviewee [DEV5] commented that *implantable devices, particularly those involving wireless devices, typically have an incredibly long and uncertain regulatory pathway in part because the FDA is "somewhat scared" of wireless technology.* Another interviewee [GENX13] noted that it can be harder to get approval for drug combinations, stating that *the rules require evidence from randomized controlled trials regarding a drug's efficacy and safety in the population for which it is intended, using outcome measures that the developer has identified. If approval is sought for a drug combination, then each of the components adds to the others in the endpoint that has been identified.* The polypill case study illustrates this point. Although each individual drug in the polypill has previously received FDA approval, and these drugs are often prescribed together, additional large-scale studies would be required to obtain approval to market a pill that combines low doses of these medications in a single tablet.

Case Study Summary

A Cardiovascular Polypill

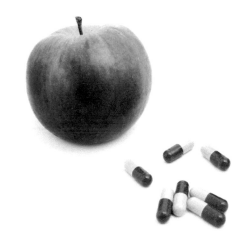

© Eldin Muratovic—Fotolia.com

The Technology: A cardiovascular "polypill" refers to a multidrug combination pill intended to reduce blood pressure and cholesterol, known risk factors for the development of cardiovascular disease. The rationale is that combining four beneficial drugs in low doses in a single pill should produce an easy and affordable way to dramatically modify cardiovascular risk. Epidemiological models suggest that widespread use of a polypill could cut the rate of heart attacks and strokes in half or more, dramatically reducing mortality, morbidity, and the associated costs of treating these conditions.

Promising But Not Rigorously Evaluated: Multiple polypills have been created over the past decade. The ingredients of the pill—three low-dose antihypertensives and a statin—are all FDA approved. Doctors frequently prescribe one or more of these pills to their patients, but they must be taken separately. The epidemiological data supporting the potential benefits of taking a polypill are impressive but largely theoretical. Several small-scale trials outside the United States have produced promising findings, but U.S. regulators consider them insufficient to establish the polypill's safety and efficacy. Additional prospective studies are under way, mostly with the support from non-U.S. governments and academic institutions.

Given the level of evidence required to secure FDA approval of new drugs in the United States and the high cost of conducting large phase III clinical trials in the United States, there is little chance that a pharmaceutical company will invest the money required to bring a cardiovascular polypill to market. The margins associated with a low-cost drug like a polypill are simply too small to provide sufficient return on investment, regardless of the pill's potentially huge societal value.

Legal Obstacles Constitute an Added Barrier to Marketability: Several patent applications have been filed, including the original one by Dr. Nicholas Wald in 2000 (GB2361186). Their existence poses an additional barrier to adoption: Once a company spends the millions of dollars required to secure regulatory approval, it could find itself in costly and protracted patent litigation.

Development Block: The cardiovascular polypill is an example of "development block." Although the technology offers the prospect of tremendous value to society in terms of health benefits per dollar spent, its pace of development is slowed by the lack of an encouraging business model. For example, many physicians like to tailor their treatments to individual patients and adjust dosage levels over time; a polypill limits their ability to do so. In sum, given the way new drugs are currently patented, regulated, and paid for in the United States, inventors sometimes cannot justify the cost required to seek regulatory approval.

No one knows how many promising drugs and devices may be languishing on the fringes of the U.S. health care marketplace. A technique called "technology foraging" is being used by the Office of Science & Technology in the U.S. Department of Homeland Security to identify existing but largely overlooked inventions that can be swiftly adopted to meet agency needs. A similar program at HHS or a large integrated delivery system might be used to identify promising health care technologies that could deliver better health at lower cost.

Another interviewee [DRUG1] mentioned the *high level of evidence required for the approval of new drugs that target common diseases, such as drugs for cardiovascular conditions. Developers are required to prove efficacy in large numbers of people.* However, extra caution by the FDA in reviewing drugs that might be used by unusually large numbers of people makes sense because the benefits of ensuring safety are proportionally larger. Moreover, the potential market rewards for such a drug will also be higher. Other interviewees emphasized what they see as an unnecessarily high level of information required for the approval of devices or drugs that are similar to products already on the market. Another side of the story is that product similarity does not imply similar safety profiles. For example, some statins (e.g., Baycol) and glitazones, which are treatments for type 2 diabetes (e.g., Rezulin), have much worse side effects than others (S. Garber, 2013, Chapter Four).

One way to reduce delays without compromising the quality of FDA reviews is to increase the number of FDA staff qualified to review applications and make decisions. "User fees"—introduced for drugs in 1992 and for medical devices in 2002—for companies applying for FDA approvals have been used to increase FDA staff. (Both kinds of fees remain in effect today.)

There is some evidence that faster approval times for drugs during the 1990s increased R&D levels of seven major U.S. drug companies by several billion dollars (Vernon et al., 2009). However, one provider who we interviewed expressed concern that the *FDA is not as careful about monitoring devices, citing the limited follow-up on complaints about robotic surgery.*

Unpredictability and Ineffective Communication Complicate the Approval Process

Concerns have also been raised about applicants' inability to predict what studies and information will be required to gain FDA approval and about ineffective communication between the FDA and product sponsors (Makower, Meer, and Denend, 2010; U.S. Government Accountability Office [GAO], 2012b, 2012c). There are reports of the FDA adding requirements for approval during the review process, as well as complaints about poor communication between the FDA and applicants concerning requirements. Reported causes of such problems include changes in FDA personnel responsible for an application and failure of key participants to attend important meetings (Makower, Meer, and Denend, 2010).

There is some indication that these problems have been somewhat mitigated since 2010 (Edney and Larkin, 2013). Nonetheless, our interviewees expressed mixed views regarding whether the situation had improved. On the device side, many of our interviewees pointed to growing uncertainty. One said that *it is becoming increasingly common for start-up device companies to have their applications rejected by the FDA and be asked to do another clinical trial* [DEV3].

FDA Caution May Be a Root Cause of Regulatory Delay

A core mission of the FDA is to ensure that products are reasonably safe before they are used by large numbers of U.S. patients. Some observers believe that the FDA's level of caution is excessive if viewed from the broader social perspective of appropriately balancing risks and benefits, particularly for certain types of products. However, there is some evidence that—as many researchers and commentators believe—user fees and quicker approvals are associated with greater post-marketing safety problems (Olson, 2008).

A leading cause of FDA caution may be political pressure from Congress, many commentators, and the public (Baciu, Stratton, and Burke, 2007; Calfee et al., 2008; Philipson and Sun, 2008). More specifically, injuries attributed to FDA-approved medical products are tangible and tend to attract substantial attention on Capitol Hill and in the press, casting the FDA in a bad light. In contrast, forgone health benefits are intangible and receive less media and congressional attention. On the other hand, as reported by a member of our expert panel, excess caution may be more attributable to FDA staff members' fear of making mistakes that would lead to deaths and serious injuries.

Thus, the FDA faces a dilemma. The agency is under pressure from those who think it moves too quickly, thus jeopardizing safety; at the same time, the agency is criticized by those who think it moves too slowly, thus denying patients quick access to good medicines. The Avastin case study provides an example of the hazards of speeding up the process. The accelerated approval of Avastin for treating metastatic breast cancer was later revoked by the FDA based on results from subsequent clinical trials. But FDA approval allowed Avastin to secure a place on a major drug compendium, thus assuring that Medicare will continue to pay for the drug's off-label use. The FDA's later revocation of its approval for the metastatic breast cancer indication (in response to results from additional trials suggesting troublesome side effects and little, if any, efficacy) did not lead Medicare to withdraw coverage of Avastin for metastatic breast cancer.

Avastin for Metastatic Breast Cancer

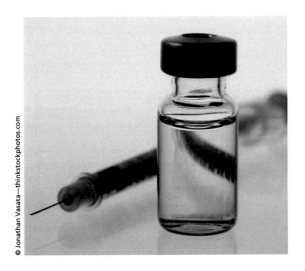

© Jonathan Vasata—thinkstockphotos.com

The Technology: Bevacizumab (brand name: Avastin) is a recombinant humanized monoclonal antibody that binds to human vascular endothelial growth factor, preventing its interaction with receptors on the surface of endothelial cells. It blocks angiogenesis, the development of new blood vessels—a process essential for cancer growth. Developed by Roche/Genentech, Avastin is widely used as an adjunctive therapy to traditional chemotherapies in the treatment of several types of cancers.

Adoption: Avastin was adopted rapidly. The first FDA-approved use for Avastin in oncology came in 2004 after a successful phase III trial in metastatic colorectal cancer, funded by Genentech (Hurwitz et al., 2004). Subsequently, FDA approvals were won for the second-line treatment of metastatic colorectal cancer (2006), non–small cell lung cancer (2006), and, later, other forms of cancer (National Cancer Institute, 2013).

E2100, the clinical trial that was cited to support initial approval for use of Avastin in metastatic breast cancer, was published in 2007 (Miller et al., 2007). The FDA's Oncologic Drugs Advisory Committee Clinical (ODAC) found the evidence weak on multiple dimensions: Patients treated with Avastin had a 5.5-month increase in *progression-free survival*, but no improvement in overall survival or quality of life. On this basis, ODAC recommended against approval. Nevertheless, the FDA granted "accelerated approval" of a metastatic breast cancer indication in early 2008; this allowed Genentech to market the drug, provided it conducted additional studies to address ODAC's concerns.

FDA Approval Later Revoked: In 2011, based on subsequent clinical trials that found only slight improvements in progression-free survival, no net gain in overall survival, and a *higher* rate of serious adverse events in patients treated with Avastin, the FDA revoked its approval for Avastin in treating metastatic breast cancer. The decision dismayed patients and oncologists who were convinced that the drug was beneficial, regardless of the scientific evidence. They loudly protested the decision.

Perverse Effects of Reimbursement Policy: The Avastin story not only highlights the dilemma posed by the pressure to quickly approve potential breakthrough drugs on the basis of "surrogate endpoints" like progression-free survival, it also illustrates various oddities in how physician-administered drugs are reimbursed. In 2003, federal law set physician reimbursement for outpatient administration of these drugs through Medicare Part B to the manufacturer's average sales price plus 6 percent and an administrative fee; this fee went into effect in 2005. While this temporarily lowered Part B drug reimbursements, of which chemotherapy drugs are the majority, it gave manufacturers a perverse incentive to compete on the basis of charging the highest price, because this encourages physicians to pick their product over equally effective but less expensive alternatives. In addition, the Social Security Act of 1993 requires that Medicare reimburse all anticancer drugs and biologics listed in certain drug compendia, even drugs that are prescribed off label. Because Avastin had secured a spot on a major drug compendium for use in metastatic breast cancer shortly before the FDA changed course, and is available for use to treat other forms of cancer, Medicare must continue to pay for its now off-label use to treat metastatic breast cancer, despite the FDA's withdrawal of regulatory approval for the metastatic breast cancer indication.

The Regulator's Dilemma: The FDA's experience with Avastin illustrates the difficult balancing act that the agency must maintain between those who think it moves too slowly and those who think it moves too quickly. The agency granted accelerated approval for Avastin's use in metastatic breast cancer on the basis of a single clinical trial using surrogate endpoints. By the time additional research determined that the drug did not increase survival or improve the quality of life for patients with this condition, the drug had built a loyal following among oncologists who profited from its use and a subgroup of patients who were convinced that it helped *them*. During the relatively brief time period that Avastin held accelerated approval, it secured a spot on major drug compendia. This ensures that Medicare must continue to pay for the drug's use to treat metastatic breast cancer even though it is now off label.

Regulatory Risk Figures Prominently in Investment and Invention Decisions

Most of the investors and inventors we interviewed mentioned "regulatory risk" as a key consideration in investment decisions. Inventors and investors seem averse to unpredictability about whether a product will be approved and how long that will take. They report that greater regulatory uncertainty tends to reduce R&D efforts and the level of investment in particular areas. As one interviewee put it, *If you are going to invest 500 million dollars in something, you need some confidence that the guidance you received from the FDA seven years ago will still apply"* [DRUG2]. Another interviewee [INVES5] reported that substantial uncertainty regarding what the FDA would require for approval of type 2 diabetes treatments made both venture capitalists and big pharmaceutical companies reluctant to invest in the area.

Regulatory uncertainty can be particularly problematic for smaller companies, *which typically start with three or four ideas but eventually have to put money behind the idea that is furthest along (even if it is not the best idea). That means the company ends up with just one shot at success. This turns out to be a really risky shot with regards to the feelings of the FDA* [INVES3].

Another interviewee contrasted the regulatory uncertainty that product inventors often experience with the regulatory clarity related to the development of HIV treatments [DRUG5], emphasizing that *the FDA made it clear what it would require for approval for HIV treatments. A great deal of antiviral research was conducted, and treatments emerged in a very limited amount of time.* Similarly, several interviewees noted that the Orphan Drug Act has eased the regulatory pathway for rare conditions and led to increased efforts in these areas.

The implications of regulatory cost and risk differ depending on the market potential of the product in question. For example, in the case of the polypill, the profit margins associated with such a low-cost drug may simply be too small to generate sufficient return on investment to sponsor the required clinical trials or to apply for FDA approval—even if swift approval were assured and the pill could potentially lead to an extremely large public health benefit.

One interviewee [DEV6] noted *that the regulatory compliance risk in some categories of medical technology makes early-stage investing more challenging.* Another [INVES3] said that *over the last five years, new investments have been going into health IT that does not require FDA approval and health care delivery—rather than drugs and devices—because of the lack of predictability in the regulatory environment.* Another interviewee [DRUG1] suggested that *some companies have gotten out of trying to develop drugs for large populations because of the high level of cost associated with the clinical trials,* despite the fact that large populations also imply larger potential market rewards.

How Regulatory Uncertainty Affects Investment and Invention

Longer times from the beginning of invention to approval for U.S. sales make investments in FDA-regulated products less attractive to inventors and their investors. Moreover, inventors and investors seem averse to regulatory risk because of unpredictability about whether a product will be approved and how long approval will take. Some drugs and devices will appear so promising to inventors and investors that they will be invented despite the FDA-related time and monetary costs and such risks. But many potential inventive efforts may be close to the margin of being unattractive to investors; as a result, these efforts might be deterred by additional regulatory delays and uncertainty that may or may not be required to ensure product safety.

The regulatory environment can also drive inventors and investors toward incremental product improvements rather than bold, high-impact ideas. As noted by one interviewee [GENX8], *the biggest impediment to high-value innovation—one that pushed developers to go in safer directions—is the difficult regulatory pathway. There's a lot of uncertainty in the industry regarding what the FDA will or won't do at any point in time.* In sum, if the delays and uncertainties associated with the FDA process are not necessary to protect public safety, then inventive efforts deterred by excess delays and uncertainty may represent a lost opportunity to increase health benefits per dollar spent.

Limited Rewards for Medical Products That Could Decrease Spending

In most U.S. industries, such as consumer electronics, competition greatly benefits consumers because sellers vie for business by offering product improvements, lower prices, or both. Customers tend to buy from sellers that provide the best value, which is a combination of price and product quality. Thus, market competition continually pressures producers to reduce their production costs and to develop and price new products to provide greater value to consumers.

In U.S. health care markets, however, competition does not serve consumers' interests nearly as well. Price competition among medical product manufacturers is limited because in many cases the market fails to adequately reward products with the potential to lower spending. As one interviewee [DEV3] described, *with medical devices, technology is priced as high as possible. Very few developers come to the United States and compete on price; it's a zero-sum game. If the market is divided between three players, you don't kill the market by coming in super cheap. Instead, you use other strategies, such as making sure opinion leaders like the product.*

It appears that in many cases U.S. health care markets fail to adequately reward inventors of products with the potential to lower spending. This failure results from three phenomena:

1. The decisions of many providers and patients exhibit little price sensitivity.
2. In many circumstances, providers have limited time horizons when they decide which products to use for which patients.
3. Decisionmaking is fragmented within many provider organizations.

Many Patients and Providers Are Fairly Insensitive to Prices

Decreased price sensitivity reduces inventors' market rewards for lowering prices and thereby reduces incentives to invent medical products that have the potential to reduce spending. As one interviewee [DRUG2] aptly put it, *drug companies focus on profits when they consider pricing of a product, and not much else. The issue is elasticity. Does lower price get us more patients?*

Payers, consumers, taxpayers, providers, and the popular press have raised concerns that prices of some drugs and devices are uncomfortably, even shockingly, high (Marshall, Cheson, and Kerr, 2013; Pollack, 2013; Rosenthal, 2013; Brill, 2013; Kliff, 2013). Most fundamentally, prices of medical products are determined by sellers seeking large financial rewards—for themselves and for their investors. When asked what factors into pricing decisions for new products, nearly all of our interviewees mentioned some variation of *what the market will bear.* What the market will bear for a new drug or device depends on a host of factors, including the severity of the medical condition(s) that the product addresses, the product's effectiveness, whether there are other products and/or services that address the same medical condition(s), and the effectiveness and prices of such substitutes. For example, the market will bear very high prices for a new drug or device that is very effective in treating a serious medical condition and has no good substitutes (such as other branded drugs in the same therapeutic class and generic drugs).

Inventors who anticipate only modest financial rewards are disadvantaged in obtaining needed financial capital from private investors. One developer (academic) said that if it were up to him [GENX13], *he'd price his new technology at a level to make an economically viable business, but as inexpensive as possible. When he described his position to venture capitalists who had approached him, they walked out the door.*

Key reasons for a lack of price sensitivity in health care include generously insured patients, FFS payment, lack of price transparency, and limitations on Medicare's ability to consider cost in coverage and payment decisions. We next discuss these reasons in turn.

Generous Health Insurance Tends to Reduce Consumers' Sensitivity to Price

About 85 percent of Americans have private or public health insurance. Those with generous insurance—by which we mean fairly low deductibles and rates of cost-sharing—are unlikely to consider price when deciding which health services to consume. This is because receiving additional services costs generously insured patients little or no out-of-pocket costs once they have exceeded their deductibles. Instead, most if not all of the extra spending they generate comes out of the pockets of others, such as other members of their insurance pools and taxpayers. Thus, when the manufacturers' price for a medical product decreases, the cost to many patients does not decrease nearly as much. As a result, when a new treatment comes on the market at a lower price than comparable treatments for a similar condition, many patients are less likely to switch to the new treatment than if they had to pay the full price out of pocket.

Most public health insurance plans are generous. For example, most Medicare enrollees are in traditional FFS Medicare. Further lowering price sensitivity for many of these enrollees, in 2012 about 9.5 million enrollees in traditional Medicare were covered by Medigap insurance plans (AHIP Coverage, 2013), which decrease deductibles and cost-sharing. Thus, we expect that most people who are covered by Medicare are fairly insensitive to price in many circumstances. Medicaid has roughly 58 million enrollees (FamiliesUSA, 2014), who also have low cost-sharing. However, roughly 50 million of them are enrolled in managed care plans, which negotiate vigorously to keep the prices they pay for drugs and devices low (Medicaid.gov, undated).

Turning to private insurance, the RAND Health Insurance Experiment, conducted during the 1970s and 1980s, investigated the price sensitivity of demand for medical care. The investigators estimated that a 10-percent increase in out-of-pocket cost of medical care would result in a 2-percent decrease in the amount of care used (Newhouse and the Insurance Experiment Group, 1993). Most more-recent econometric estimates are in the range of the RAND estimate, including demand for prescription drugs (Chandra, Cutler, and Song, 2012, pp. 408–409). Presumably, most consumers are insensitive to price changes that do not affect their out-of-pocket costs.

Many privately insured Americans have generous insurance, but many do not. According to the Kaiser Family Foundation and Health Research & Educational Trust (2013), during 2013 almost 150 million nonelderly people were covered by employer-sponsored insurance (ESI) plans, the generosity of which differs substantially across plans. Moreover, in 2011 about 11.5 million Americans were enrolled in high-deductible health plans (HDHPs), which are required to have deductibles of as least $1,200 and $2,400 for individual and families, respectively (Kulkarni, 2012), and annual deductibles of $2,000 to $4,000 are not uncommon. Thus, health care spending for most services delivered to HDHP enrollees is entirely out of pocket until they exceed their deductibles; such enrollees will tend to have fairly high price sensitivity until their deductibles are reached.

It appears that recent trends have been reducing the number of Americans with generous insurance. For example, the prevalence (and generosity) of employer-sponsored health insurance is declining, and the prevalence of HDHPs has been increasing (Carrns, 2013). Moreover, changes due to the ACA will also reduce the number of Americans with generous insurance. First, the 40-percent excise tax on especially generous ESI plans (sometimes called "Cadillac plans") instituted by the ACA (to begin in 2018) will tend to reduce the number of Americans with generous health insurance ("Health Policy Brief: Excise Tax on 'Cadillac' Plans," 2013). Second, cost-sharing rates in the bronze and silver plans that can be purchased in the health insurance exchanges created by the ACA will be fairly high: 40 and 30 percent, respectively. Even though lower-income enrollees who purchase insurance from these exchanges will be eligible for tax credits—which are a form of premium support as that term was used by Aaron and Reischauer (1995)—the fairly high cost-sharing rates will give enrollees strong incentives to avoid unnecessary care and to seek lower-cost providers for the care they receive. (Also see Aaron, 2011.)

Another important factor tends to increase price sensitivity for drugs that patients self-administer. In particular, many large buyers of drugs—such as large health plans, employers, PBMs, and hospital chains—have market power, and they use it to negotiate lower prices from drug companies. Most often, purchasers offer more preferred placement on formularies in exchange for lower prices, and negotiations tend to reduce prices from manufacturers, especially when there are several competing drugs in a class (Scott Morton and Kyle, 2012). However, prices paid by large drug purchasers will tend to lower spending only to the degree that the lower prices are passed on to consumers.

Fee-for-Service Payment Also Tends to Reduce Price Sensitivity

When consumers delegate service decisions to their physicians, as they often do, the question becomes the extent to which *physician* choices are sensitive to manufacturers' product prices. A major factor tending to reduce the price sensitivity of physicians is FFS payment, which is still widely used by Medicare and many private insurers and rewards physicians who provide more services, whether or not they are truly beneficial. And when physicians perform more procedures, they make more money. (See the implantable cardioverter-defibrillator case study summary later in this chapter.)

Lack of Price Transparency Also Reduces Price Sensitivity

There is another reason that demand for health care is less sensitive to price than it would otherwise be. Consumers and physicians who make utilization decisions and hospitals that make purchasing decisions are often uninformed about the spending implications of their choices (GAO, 2012a; Gawande, 2012; Rosenberg, 2013). Even if they want to choose the least expensive option, they are unable to compare prices, or doing so is dauntingly time-consuming. One interviewee described the health care industry as one *where you don't know what it's going to cost you until you get the bill—we need more transparency so consumers can make smarter decisions. You do more research on what car or refrigerator you'll buy than you do on health care decisions* [DEV6].

Medicare Is Not Allowed to Consider Costs in Coverage and Reimbursement Decisions

By law, Medicare is required to cover and pay for products and services that are "reasonable and necessary" for diagnosis or treatment, and cost is not a factor in determining what is reasonable and necessary (Neumann, Kamae, and Palmer, 2008; Neumann and Chambers, 2012). As a result, Medicare is obliged to pay for some medical technologies that are not cost-effective (Chambers, Neumann, and Buxton, 2010), even when there are equally effective options that are less expensive. However, some evidence suggests that cost-effectiveness information may play a role in some national coverage decisions (Chambers et al., 2011).

Over the years, Medicare has taken a number of steps to try to reduce program costs. Some of these initiatives, such as the prospective payment systems that have been implemented in many service settings, have been successful. Payment to Medicare Advantage (Part C) plans—which now cover 29 percent of Medicare beneficiaries—is capitated. In addition, the ACA also mandates a number of cost-reducing demonstrations: ACOs with shared cost savings, bundling of more comprehensive episodes of care, and competitive pricing for medical supplies. Demonstrations are being conducted by CMS's Innovation Center (CMS, undated [a]) and the Patient-Centered Outcomes Research Institute (PCORI) to support its mission "to answer questions important to patients and meaningfully involve patients and others across the healthcare community at all stages of the research process" (PCORI, 2014). Moreover, prices paid to drug manufacturers for enrollees in Medicare Part D drug plans—which are administered by private health insurers—are negotiated by these insurers, who use preferred formulary placement as the carrot.

In some cases, Medicare's prohibition against considering cost-effectiveness may undermine the value of services provided to Medicare enrollees. To make matters worse, private payers often follow CMS's lead in determining their coverage policies and the structure of their payment policies (such as use of prospective payments), although they do not necessarily use Medicare payment rates generally or rates for new technologies. For example, regarding devices, Medicare's "decisions and methods are followed by most private payers" (Zenios, Makower, and Yock, 2010, p. 507). One interviewee [COV3] said the *conventional wisdom is that private payers followed Medicare's lead on coverage,* although he was not aware of any systematic evidence of this. Another insurer we interviewed [COV4] said that his organization did *closely watch what CMS does, but those decisions are not the final determinant.* Thus, to the extent that some Medicare policies undermine value for services provided to Medicare enrollees, the policies may also undermine value for services provided to many enrollees in private health insurance plans.

Limited Time Horizons and Fragmented Decisionmaking

In many instances, the individuals or organizations making a decision to use (or not use) a particular health care product do not reap the full financial benefits (including future avoided costs) of that use. This phenomenon affects a wide range of medical technologies—but seems particularly important for diagnostics, treatments for chronic conditions, and preventive services—as well as the adoption of HIT. (See the EHR case study summary.) When limited time horizons and fragmented decisionmaking are factors, the demand for medical products that could help reduce spending will tend to be lower than if the entities that make purchasing decisions were able to capture all of the benefits of the lower spending.

Electronic Health Records

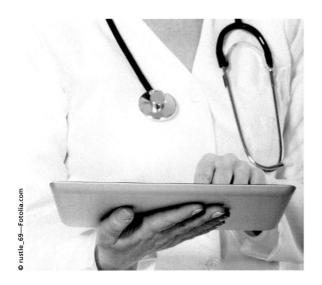

© rustle_69—Fotolia.com

The Technology: Electronic health records (EHRs) include a variety of medical documentation systems "generally focused on medical care," including patient information, diagnoses, procedure codes, and medications.

Adoption: EHRs were envisioned as early as the 1950s, with the testing of computer-based medical histories. Development of early medical information systems occurred in the 1960s and 1970s, with financial support from federal agencies, some large hospital systems, and professional associations. Creation of health maintenance organizations and their need to document care drove early adoption of EHRs and broadened uptake, but most health care systems self-funded their EHRs. Multiple studies project large potential benefits from adoption based on optimistic assumptions regarding uptake, interoperability, and implementation.

The HITECH Act Offered Financial Incentives for Adoption: Through the Health Information Technology for Economic and Clinical Health (HITECH) Act, a provision of the American Recovery and Reinvestment Act of 2009, the federal government injected billions of dollars in incentives into the health care system to spur adoption and "meaningful use" of EHRs. To date, roughly 55 percent of eligible physicians and nearly 4,000 hospitals have taken advantage of the HITECH Act's incentives.

Multiple Barriers to Adoption Remain: Rapid adoption of EHRs has been hindered by a variety of factors, including a fragmented marketplace, changing federal incentives, provider uncertainty about the regulatory landscape, concerns about limited usability, and a general lack of interoperability between systems. Uptake has been particularly slow among smaller hospitals and physician groups, and cost remains a concern. Many providers perceive that payers and vendors reap the economic benefits of an EHR, while providers bear the cost of implementation.

Although connectivity—the ability to share data through a health information exchange—was an important requirement in the HITECH Act, rules issued by the HHS to guide implementation of the act watered down this requirement. The practical effect of this policy decision was to promote adoption of existing platforms, rather than encourage the development of interoperable and inter-connected systems. Provisions in the ACA will raise the bar for physicians and hospitals to qualify for federal incentives in 2014. If implemented as drafted, they will enhance interoperability and should substantially increase the value of EHRs to health care pro-viders and patients.

Current Major Players—VistA and Epic: To illustrate how market forces and public policy shape adoption of EHRs, consider two of the largest and most influential EHRs in the United States today—VistA and Epic.

VistA, the Veterans' Health Information Systems and Technol-ogy Architecture, has been implemented throughout the Veterans Health Administration. Intensively studied since its inception, VistA has been credited with reducing costs, improving patient care, and enhancing clinical outcomes in the VA health care system (Brown et al., 2003; Rundle, 2001). Because its architecture is designed to enable the ready retrieval and analysis of clinical data, it has proven to be a powerful tool for quality improvement and health services research. VistA incorporated, and in some instances pioneered, sev-eral useful features, including computerized order entry, electronic prescribing, bar code medication administration, and embedded clinical guidelines.

VistA's success has been attributed in large part to the collaborative nature of its development. Clinicians and information technology (IT) experts worked together to design its user interfaces and patient record system. Equally if not more important, because VistA is built on a standard code and maintains data-sharing capability between sites, it is fully interoperable within the VA.

Despite its known strengths and many favorable reviews by physicians, VistA has not been enthusiastically embraced by the private market. Medsphere, a company created to market OpenVista (a version of VistA adapted for commercial use) and related products, has a modest foothold in the market, but most hospitals and providers have purchased commercial products that they believe are better designed to meet their needs, particularly billing.

Epic is a privately held company that develops, installs, supports, and owns its proprietary technology. Among Epic's 260-plus clients are most of the United States' elite academic medical centers. Epic does customized installations for each client, allowing health care systems to tailor Epic's applications and functionality to meet their own needs. But customizability limits Epic's interoperability between sites and hinders its capacity to communicate with other EHRs. Certain aspects of Epic's architecture, including its reliance on free text entry, hinder its utility as a health services research tool.

Notwithstanding these limitations, Epic is highly successful commercially. According to a recent article in *Forbes* magazine, "By next year [2013], 127 million patients or nearly 40% of the U.S. population will have its medical information stored in an Epic digital record" (Moukheiber, 2013).

The EHR "Productivity Paradox": When other U.S. industries adopted IT in the 1970s and 1980s, productivity growth initially fell. However, when these industries redesigned their IT systems to make them more usable by employees and customers and redesigned work processes to take advantage of IT's capabilities, productivity soared. Health care has yet to take a similar approach. It is not known how use of EHRs in the United States will evolve, but two points are clear: (1) EHRs are here to stay, and (2) how they are designed and employed will profoundly influence the quality, efficiency, and cost of American health care for decades to come.

Often the health benefits from using a drug, device, or HIT are not realized until years in the future, at which time the patient is likely to be covered by a different insurer. When this is the case, the later insurer will obtain the financial benefits associated with the (long-delayed) health benefits. For example, consider effective hypertension medications or cholesterol-lowering drugs. Use of such drugs for patients enrolled in private health plans may prevent heart attacks that would have occurred years later when many of these patients will be enrolled in Medicare. Thus, part of the social benefit of the decision accrues to Medicare, not to the insurer or provider who paid for the drug.

One interviewee [PROV3] described the challenges faced by payers in fully accounting for value: *Patient populations in insurance plans are not there for life. The average duration of membership in a Medicaid program is eight months. How do you manage value measurably? We may not see an effect, but **someone** will.* Another interviewee told us that [DRUG 5] *Payers tend to have a short-term perspective. A life saved in the future provides no financial value. Payers do not benefit from cancer prevention through screening.* In the context of preventive services, some of which could decrease spending, another interviewee [GENX1] reported, *when you look at preventive services, the reason that developers are deterred or discouraged from creating high-value technology that lowers overall spending revolves around reimbursement . . . . we can't set future value to justify the price of preventive services. There's no market incentive.*

In addition, when a health system is siloed—i.e., decisionmakers consider the costs and benefits for only part of an organization—few, if any, decisionmakers account for benefits or costs that accrue outside of their silos. One interviewee described the problem as follows: [GENX12] *Let's say you have a new diagnostic technique and it gives you a huge benefit in timely diagnosis of a very contagious disease versus, say, a baseline and slower technique. Those making the buy decision [in the lab] are compartmentalized. What determines the purchase is the profit/loss assessment for their department [the lab], the price per unit and running cost in the lab component. They have no ability to analyze or account for benefits that accrue to other departments [such as the ER] from the time advantage in triaging the patient. That will be picked up in the profit and loss statement of another disconnected unit. There's little ability to do longitudinal holistic decisionmaking and evaluation of cost-benefit.*

Limited time horizons and fragmented decisionmaking have played substantial roles in the development, adoption, and use of HIT, as highlighted in our EHR case study. Several studies projected large potential benefits from EHR adoption based on optimistic assumptions regarding uptake, interoperability, and implementation. The potential benefits of well-implemented EHRs extend well beyond the providers who must make the investment in the technology and bear the costs of implementation. As one interviewee described [HIT1], *Payers could potentially use data to better target reimbursements; developers could access data from EHRs to study the effectiveness to treatments.* Instead, HIT providers have developed business models that respond to organizational pressures of potential customers by creating EHRs that provide direct benefits to the organization making the investments, not just payers downstream.

The U.S. government has tried to shape the market for HIT by offering monetary incentives for adopting EHRs and using them to exchange information and improve the quality of care. The Health Information Technology (HITECH) Act, which is part of the American Recovery and Reinvestment Act of 2009, provided $19 billion for HIT investment, including payments to providers for adopting certified EHRs demonstrating "meaningful use." The MU criteria have been rolled out in stages. The first stage focused on the electronic capture of health information by the provider and electronic access to health information by patients. The second stage focused on enabling and promoting the exchange of electronic health information among providers and between patients and providers. The third stage is pending and is expected to focus on the use of electronic information to improve the quality of care.

But despite satisfying the MU criteria, most systems have very little capability to share information; i.e., they have poor interoperability capabilities that greatly reduce their value (Executive Office of the President, 2010; Hare, 2010). Moreover, many providers are dissatisfied with their EHR systems (Eastwood, 2013). In an effort to overcome or mitigate the interoperability problems, in March 2013 several providers of EHRs formed a nonprofit organization called CommonWell Health Alliance (CommonWell Health Alliance, 2014; Herper, 2013).

Inadequate Rewards for Products That Decrease Spending

We have no quantitative empirical information about the average market rewards for inventing products that tend to decrease spending relative to those that increase it; such information would be extremely challenging—and perhaps impossible—to develop. But we do believe that the theoretical arguments suggesting inadequate market rewards for such products are strong and deserve to be seriously considered.

We are not suggesting that market rewards are never adequate to spur invention of products that would tend to decrease spending. In fact, me-too drugs are likely to help reduce drug acquisition costs for such large buyers as large health systems, hospital chains, and PBMs because they increase such buyers' bargaining power relative to drug manufacturers. To the extent that savings are passed on to consumers rather than being added to profits of large drug purchasers, me-too drugs will tend to decrease U.S. spending on health care. But such examples may be more the exception than the rule. For example, health economist David Cutler—a leading proponent of the view that, averaged over all technologies, health benefits of new technologies have been worth the extra spending—has written, "In some cases, new technologies replace more expensive existing treatments and thus save money, but this is rare" (Cutler, 2004, p. 71).

Perhaps most important, when the market rewards for inventing products that are likely to decrease spending are inadequate, there may be public or private policy initiatives that could improve the financial attractiveness of inventing these products.

Implications for Inventors and Investors

Weak market demand for medical products that could decrease spending limits the market rewards for inventing new products that have such potential and, as a result, limits incentives for inventing such products. Little price sensitivity of many patients and providers, limited time horizons, and fragmented decisionmaking play roles in this regard. The cardiovascular polypill is an example of a product that has great potential to increase value but is stalled by low potential profits.

In sum, reduced financial rewards due to several institutional features of U.S. health care make many inventors and most private investors less willing to support the invention of medical products that could reduce spending. As a result, such products will be less likely to be invented and be offered for sale in the United States.

Treatment Creep

The value of a treatment or diagnostic test depends on the health benefits it provides for the patients who use it. Broadly speaking, treatment creep is defined as the use of a medical product for patients other than the originally intended users. Some forms of treatment creep can be socially desirable. For example, as physicians become more experienced with and adept at performing a procedure, it might become appropriate for more patients, such as those who are frail.

In contrast, undesirable treatment creep occurs when a medical technology that provides substantial health benefits to a particular subpopulation is used for other patients for whom the health benefits are much smaller or completely absent (Bentley et al., 2008, p. 644). Our case study of the implantable cardioverter-defibrillator (ICD) illustrates this phenomenon.

Case Study Summary

Implantable Cardioverter-Defibrillator

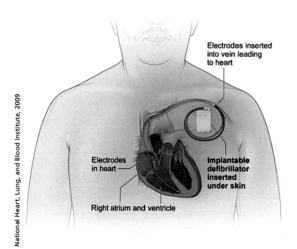

Electrodes inserted into vein leading to heart

Electrodes in heart

Implantable defibrillator inserted under skin

Right atrium and ventricle

National Heart, Lung, and Blood Institute, 2009

The Technology: An implantable cardioverter-defibrillator (ICD) is an implantable device consisting of a small pulse generator (roughly half the size of a smartphone) and one or more thin wire leads threaded through large blood vessels into the heart. ICDs are designed to sense a life-threatening cardiac arrhythmia and automatically provide a dose of direct current (DC) electricity to jolt the patient's heart back to normal.

Originally, defibrillators delivered jolts of DC electricity through external paddles placed on the patient's chest. The first internal defibrillator was surgically implanted in 1980 at the Johns Hopkins Medical Center by Dr. Levi Watkins and Vivien

Thomas, pioneering African American medical researchers. In 1985, the FDA approved the first implantable defibrillator. The first transvenous defibrillator lead was approved in 1993.

Initial Adoption for Secondary Prevention: ICDs were first used for secondary prevention of sudden cardiac death. Patients in this group were defined as having survived a prior cardiac arrest or an episode of sustained ventricular tachycardia. Trials published between 1997 and 2000 proved the lifesaving worth of the technology and formed the rationale for the American Heart Association guidelines for use of ICDs in secondary sudden cardiac death prevention.

Expansion to Primary Prevention: Subsequently, a series of costly clinical trials sponsored by public-private partnerships provided evidence of the value of ICDs in primary prevention for patients with and without ischemic heart disease. The Sudden Cardiac Death in Heart Failure Trial published in 2005 serves as the basis for current guidelines and payment coverage in this population.

Not All Groups Benefit: These trials also identified subgroups for whom ICD therapy provides little or no benefit, such as patients who are undergoing bypass surgery or in the early period following a heart attack, the first three months following coronary revascularization, severe heart failure (New York Heart Association Class IV), and those with newly diagnosed heart failure. In these cases, there is no evidence that implanting an ICD increases survival or improves the patient's quality of life.

Diffusion Enabled by Medicare's Decisions: Because ICDs are costly, their diffusion has been largely driven by whether or not public and private payers will pay for the technology. Because private insurance companies generally follow Medicare's lead, CMS has played an important role in enabling ICD diffusion.

Medicare's decision to cover use for secondary prevention was relatively straightforward, and Medicare issued its first coverage decision in 1986, one year after the FDA approved ICDs. The decision regarding whether to expand coverage of ICD therapy to primary prevention was much more controversial because the benefits were less clear and the financial consequences were much greater. Nevertheless, as more clinical trial results were reported, CMS expanded coverage.

A pivotal decision was reached in 2003, when Medtronic Inc. released preliminary data from a trial that included patients with ejection fractions (volume of blood pumped from the heart with each heart beat) of 30 percent (about 60 percent of normal function) or less due to either nonischemic or ischemic heart disease. The company pressed CMS to expand coverage to include this larger group of patients. CMS consulted with other ICD manufacturers and with professional societies and elicited public comment on multiple occasions. Ultimately, CMS determined that ICDs were "reasonable and necessary" for primary prevention of sudden cardiac death (SCD) in this much larger group of patients. Implantations grew by 20 to 30 percent annually between 1985, the year ICDs secured FDA approval, and the mid-2000s. Today, primary prevention accounts for four out of every five ICD implants.

To ensure that its decision produced the benefits promised by manufacturers and experts, CMS specified that it would reimburse providers only if patients receiving an ICD for primary prevention were enrolled in an FDA-approved clinical trial, a clinical trial managed by CMS, or another organization's approved treatment registry (McClellan and Tunis, 2005). (The policy, known as "coverage with evidence development," is similar to the FDA's "accelerated approval" process.)

Health Impact: Numerous trials have shown that ICDs significantly reduce rates of death from SCD when implanted in properly selected patients. However, there are no published studies that quantify how ICDs have changed the overall incidence of SCD.

In addition, ICDs are often implanted in patients who are less likely to benefit. Based on clinical trials, the American Heart Association recommends against implanting ICDs in certain clinical contexts and for certain groups. Unfortunately, clinicians often ignore this guidance. Among 25,000 patients enrolled in the National Cardiovascular Data Registry's ICD Registry, nearly one in four received an ICD for a non–evidence-based indication.

Cost-Effectiveness: ICDs are not risk-free: An ICD may inappropriately deliver one or more painful shocks. The site of implantation can become infected. ICD leads can fracture. Cost-effectiveness studies estimate that the cost of implanting an ICD for primary prevention of SCD is between $34,000 and $72,000 per quality-adjusted life year (QALY) gained, a number in the general ballpark of treating end-stage renal disease, which Medicare uses as a reference point for cost-effectiveness comparisons. However, the analyses do not consider the cost of potential complications, such as infection or inappropriate shocks, or their effect on a patient's quality of life. In addition, the studies assumed implantation of a single-chamber ICD. Today, more than two-thirds of patients receive a far more expensive dual-chamber device, although such devices have not been found to improve outcomes and are associated with more complications.

"Treatment Creep": The rapid diffusion of ICD technology was likely driven by a series of positive clinical trials; the encouragement of manufacturers; and, most importantly, the willingness of CMS to progressively expand the population of patients who qualify for coverage. Professional societies and groups have attempted to place reasonable boundaries on the use of ICDs. However, such guidelines are often ignored.

CMS's *coverage with evidence development* policy makes ongoing assessment of ICDs possible. With increasing data on the effectiveness of ICDs, cardiologists can provide more individualized assessments of likely benefits and risks. In *carefully selected* patients, implantation of an ICD saves lives at a price per QALY in line with other costly but widely accepted life-sustaining technologies, such as renal dialysis. The challenge with ICDs and other high-technology devices is to limit their use to patients who are most likely to benefit and discourage their implantation in patients who are unlikely to benefit from this expensive and potentially hazardous technology.

In some cases, use of a technology can even be harmful to health. An example is CT scanning, the use of which is growing rapidly. CT scans subject the human body to between 150 and 1,100 times the radiation of a conventional X-ray. It has been estimated that increasing use of head, chest, abdominal, and pelvic CT scans—one-third of which appear not to be "justified by medical need"—may be responsible for as many as 2 percent of all cancer cases in the United States (Brenner and Hall, 2007).

Treatment creep also describes situations in which the risk of a mistaken diagnosis can lead patients to undergo a painful or risky treatment that is unnecessary or unproven to work for their problem. For example, the rapid uptake and dissemination of PSA screening triggered a marked increase in the diagnosis and treatment of prostate cancers, many of which would have remained clinically occult or produced indolent disease that would have never harmed the patient. The risk of mistaken diagnosis pertains to other cancers as well (Esserman, Thompson, and Reid, 2013; Orenstein, 2013).

Manufacturers Can Promote Low-Value Use

Manufacturers engage in permissible practices that can sway physicians, patients, and payers to use products in ways that do not provide good value—for example, manufacturers may provide support for research studies that are not up to FDA standards (Stafford, 2008; Pstay and Ray, 2008; Mello, Studdert, and Brennan, 2009). These dynamics are illustrated in the ICD case study, where the rapid diffusion of ICD technology was driven by favorable clinical trials on narrow populations, the encouragement of manufacturers, and, most importantly, the willingness of CMS to progressively expand the population of patients who qualify for Medicare coverage for the device. Professional societies and groups have attempted to place reasonable boundaries on the use of ICDs, but such guidance is often ignored.

Physicians and patients can be easy to sway. When a diagnostic test is available, doctors—partly in response to concerns about medical malpractice claims (Carrier, Pham, and Rich, 2013)—and patients alike want to know what condition they may be dealing with, even when there may be no treatment once it is diagnosed. As described by one interviewee [COV3], *There is a lot of demand for extra testing to rule things out. We want a better picture or diagnosis, even if that information has no value in terms of targeting treatment. There is a lot of diagnostic use going after small risks. People want to know, and the negative consequences may outweigh the benefits.* Clinicians often emphasize the potential benefits of a treatment but fail to inform patients about potential risks or side effects.

PSA testing to screen for prostate cancer is a case in point. (See the prostate-specific antigen case study summary.) This blood test has been heavily promoted for years, and Medicare coverage is mandated under federal law. Although PSA testing boosts health care spending for follow-up testing, biopsies, treatments, and management of treatment-related side effects, there is little evidence that the test has reduced death rates caused by prostate cancer.

Case Study Summary

Prostate-Specific Antigen

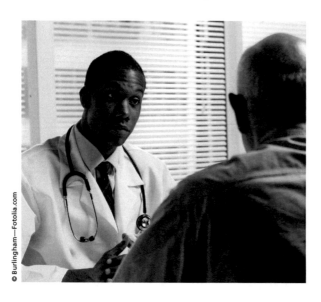

© Burlingham—Fotolia.com

The Technology: Prostate-specific antigen (PSA) is a protein secreted by the prostate gland. Low levels of PSA are present in the serum of all men, but elevated serum PSA levels correlate with a higher likelihood of having prostate cancer.

Adoption: PSA testing was first used in the late 1980s to monitor prostate cancer treatment; the FDA approved PSA testing for prostate cancer screening in 1994. Even before approval,

PSA testing became widespread among cancer-free men. Rapid implementation led to a sharp spike in the prevalence of detected disease, not because incidence of prostate cancer was rising, but because the test detected many localized cancers in otherwise asymptomatic men.

PSA screening was enthusiastically supported by professional organizations and the public; the Balanced Budget Act of 1997 mandated federal coverage of the test. Subsequently, CMS approved PSA testing in a national coverage determination process, effective January 1, 2000. Since then, frequency of PSA testing has nearly doubled. Pharmaceutical firms and some patient groups lobbied vigorously to promote PSA use. Many continue to do so.

Studies Have Determined That Widespread Screening Causes More Harm Than Good: Despite PSA screening's initial promise, multiple studies in the United States and in Europe have found that it does not reduce prostate cancer–specific mortality. Moreover, screening is associated with substantial harms caused by over-diagnosis and the complications that can occur from aggressive treatment.

Despite Official Recommendation Against Its Use, Medicare Must Cover PSA Testing: Based on unfavorable findings, in 2012 the United States Preventive Services Task Force recommended *against* routine PSA screening for prostate cancer because the harms of screening outweigh the potential benefits. However, because federal law has not been changed, Medicare must still pay for the test's use, as well as for the subsequent biopsies, surgical procedures, nonsurgical treatments, and complications that these procedures can cause.

Unintended Consequences: When PSA testing was invented, it was hoped that it could detect cases of prostate cancer at a time when definitive treatment could be curative. Rapid dissemination of the technology triggered a surge in diagnoses, biopsies, and treatment of hidden prostate cancers, many of which would have caused no trouble during the patients' life spans. Since then, studies have determined that broad-based PSA testing has little impact on overall mortality from prostate cancer. It has, however, boosted health care spending and lowered the quality of life of individuals who are living with various complications of overly aggressive treatment or the anxiety of knowing they have cancer—even if, had it remained undetected, it may have never bothered them over the course of their lives.

Defensive Medicine Is a Form of Treatment Creep

Medical malpractice laws hold clinicians financially liable for patient injuries caused by negligent care. It is unknown how much these laws contribute to patient safety, and many argue that there are better ways to promote patient safety.

There is no doubt, however, about the *existence*—as distinct from the magnitude—of a value-decreasing effect of medical malpractice laws and litigation. In particular, exposure to liability lawsuits undoubtedly leads some physicians to engage in "defensive medicine"—care that will not benefit patients and would not be delivered if it were not for clinicians' concerns about avoiding litigation. Such services include diagnostic testing, surgical procedures, and drug prescribing that provide low value and increase spending.

The extent of defensive medicine is unknown. Surveys of physicians indicate that they themselves engage in this behavior or that they believe the practice is widespread (Studdert et al., 2005; Bishop, Federman, and Keyhani, 2010; Sethi et al., 2012). Efforts to statistically link exposure to medical malpractice to wasteful care, however, have typically estimated fairly small impacts (Sloan and Shadle, 2009; Thomas, Ziller, and Thayer, 2010).

Off-Label Use of Medical Products Is Widespread, but Health Effects Are Unknown

FDA approval is required for the sale and use of a prescription drug or medical device in the United States. Such approvals are based on human (clinical) and other studies assessing the benefits and risks of drugs or devices in treating a particular condition, which are detailed on the product's FDA-regulated label. However, physicians are—as matters of law and policy—free to use drugs and devices as they and their patients see fit, including for what is called "off-label" use—that is, for conditions that have not been approved by the FDA. Physicians often prescribe off label, usually without any supporting evidence that the use of the drug or device will benefit the patient (Radley, Finkelstein, and Stafford, 2006), including orphan drugs (drugs intended to treat rare conditions; Kesselheim et al., 2012).

There are legal restrictions on how drug and device manufacturers promote (e.g., advertise) their products for off-label use (Mello, Studdert, and Brennan, 2009). But several of our interviewees emphasized that *off-label use is widespread/ubiquitous, and there are little or no data about its implications for health or for spending. Many clinicians don't understand what uses have and have not been studied once a technology is on the market, and few read the warning labels* (DEV2). Clinician and patient preferences to use the latest, cutting-edge technology are often accommodated, even in cases in which use of the technology has low value because a less costly treatment provides comparable health benefits or because the patient is not sick enough, or is too sick, to benefit.

It Is Difficult to Control Undesirable Instances of Off-Label Use

Public and private insurers could refuse to pay for off-label or inappropriate use—and, in fact, this is common according to coverage rules; however, in practice, effective enforcement of such restrictions is rare. Although some payers do try to exert such controls, one interviewee emphasized that *every time a plan does these things, it costs money. There are administrative expenses to get at this problem* [COV4]. Moreover, Medicare rules explicitly allow payment for off-label use for cancer treatments (and a handful of other specialty drugs) as long as they are reported to be appropriate for the clinical situation in one or more specified compendia (Tillman et al., 2009; Bach, 2009). (See the Avastin case study summary earlier in this chapter.)

To the extent that private insurers enforce restrictions on off-label use, they appear to be largely focused on cases where extremely expensive treatments are being used to address conditions that do not pose serious health risks. Relatively expensive imaging technologies provide examples. In particular, it is widely believed that CT, magnetic resonance imaging (MRI), and positron-emission tomography (PET) can have very large health benefits relative to alternative technologies in selected circumstances, but they are often used in situations where the health benefits are small or patients are harmed (Chandra and Skinner, 2012).

One interviewee [COV3] suggested that payers are trying to manage utilization of drugs and devices more aggressively than they have in the past. *Payers are doing this more and more and have better capacity with data systems to support these efforts. They'd like to target those most likely to benefit defined by clinical characteristics. . . Their ability to do this depends on the provider and payer data systems. It also varies across payers and patient groups.* Another interviewee suggested that *lack of data on utilization and patient conditions can impede utilization management. Simply looking at claims data is insufficient* [COV4].

An alternative to payment restrictions and monitoring is a tiered pricing or tiered reimbursement system, where the amount that patients pay for a particular treatment and/or the amount providers are paid depends on the diagnosis; this is an example of value-based insurance design (Fendrick, Smith, and Chernew, 2010; University of Michigan Center for Value-Based Insurance Design, 2013). One interviewee noted that this concept is *easy to say but hard to implement* [GENX11]. Among the challenges are dealing with treatments where the value varies across groups of patients—*how do you handle a drug that's lifesaving for a small subset of patients* [GENX11]?

Treatment creep is encouraged by FFS payment arrangements in which treating more patients leads to higher revenues, and in many instances higher profits, for health care providers. Moreover, a lack of sound evidence about the appropriate patient population for a technology (Newhouse, 2002; Chandra, Cutler, and Song, 2012; Chandra and Skinner, 2012) leaves much room for principled disagreement about the likely health benefits from using a particular technology for a particular patient. Such instances of "gray-area medicine" provide wide scope for financial incentives to result in low-value utilization (Chandra, Cutler, and Song, 2012). The growing use of ICDs is a case in point.

Treatment Creep Can Substantially Affect Incentives for Innovators

Because treatment creep is fairly common and has substantial financial implications, this phenomenon is likely a major consideration in shaping the incentives of product inventors and investors and, in turn, their decisions about which potential new medical products will and will not receive substantial investments. For example, one interviewee [DRUG2] indicated that *companies will sometimes focus on one population to get over regulatory hurdles and then shift the focus for longer-term marketing* [DRUG2]. This strategy is predicated on a manufacturer's expectation that once FDA approval for even a narrow indication is secured, use can be expanded to indications that are not approved by the FDA.

On the payment side, one interviewee noted that a *manufacturer may obtain a payment rate for a technology introduced to treat a rare medical condition; as use of the technology expands beyond the original population, however, the high payment rate may not be reduced.* For small companies in particular, the revenue generated through the initial (smaller) market can be used to further expand the market—making an otherwise unviable business strategy viable or even lucrative [DRUG2].

To the extent that treatment creep into low-value utilization provides substantial rewards for inventors and investors, it tends to encourage invention of products that deliver less value at the expense of efforts to invent ones that are likely to help further our policy goals.

Medical Arms Race

The "medical arms race" refers to an environment in which health care providers compete for business by offering new high-tech services rather than by lowering prices. This strategy relies on two widely held provider and patient beliefs: New technology is better than old, and expensive technology is better than inexpensive. (The fact that hospitals and other providers advertise the availability of high-tech treatments to patients—on radio and billboards, for example—provides evidence that many patients prefer high-tech treatments.) When these beliefs are erroneous—and they sometimes are—they drive demand for expensive new technologies and products above and beyond what would be warranted by their true clinical advantages over alternative medical interventions. This is not to deny that in some instances medical arms races could be socially beneficial—for example, when a new high-tech treatment provides good value relative to alternatives. Our concern—and the focus of the present discussion—is medical arms races that are socially undesirable and what might be done to mitigate their detrimental effects on spending and value.

The Classical Medical Arms Race

The nature of the medical arms race has evolved over the past several decades. The classic form involved hospitals in a local health care market trying to increase their patient volume by adopting cutting-edge medical technologies—often in the form of expensive medical equipment—in order to induce community physicians to practice in and admit their patients to those hospitals. The first systematic empirical evidence related to the classical medical arms race showed that hospital costs in more-competitive hospital markets tended to be higher than in less-competitive markets (Robinson and Luft, 1987). The interpretation of this pattern was that—unlike many other markets in which price competition tends to lower costs and prices—in many instances hospitals competed for physicians and patients on perceived quality (which may or may not reflect true quality).

The medical arms race was attenuated during the mid-1980s through the mid-1990s, a period during which managed care and health maintenance organizations (HMOs) "owned the patients" and used the threat of selective contracting to bargain with providers. As a result, hospitals that wanted to be in an insurer's network competed for patients by accepting lower payment rates, which put downward pressure on costs (Keeler, Melnick, and Zwanziger, 1999; Melnick and Keeler, 2007; Devers, Brewster, and Casalino, 2003).

The New Medical Arms Race
Since the mid-1990s, the managed care backlash and the growth of multihospital systems has greatly reduced the bargaining power of health plans, and a new form of the medical arms race and non-price competition has appeared (Devers, Brewster, and Casalino, 2003; Brennan, Bodenheimer, and Pham, 2006; Melnick and Keeler, 2007). Hospitals now compete among themselves and with other kinds of facilities. Much of this competition involves "specialty service lines" that are organized in various ways and focus on, for example, cardiac, oncology, or orthopedic care. This new medical arms race involves competition for patients through physician choices and by advertising directly to consumers (Brennan, Bodenheimer, and Pham, 2006).

Patients tend to assume that newer, more expensive technology is more effective (Korobkin, 2012). When it comes to high-tech screening and diagnostic equipment, patients are especially apt to lean toward new technology. Even when there is no evidence of the technology's superiority, patients view limitations on its use as an effort on the part of payers to save money (Schleifer and Rothman, 2012). Moreover, the spending implications of technologies that increase cost are of little, if any, concern to well-insured patients because most or all of the extra spending will be paid for by others.

Expensive and Controversial Medical Equipment Remains Prominent
The surgical robot exemplifies both the classical and new medical arms race. The availability of robotic surgery is used to attract physicians and patients to a facility even in the absence of evidence that robotic surgery is better than traditional treatments. As described by one interviewee [DEV3], *marketing robotic surgery to hospitals for use in prostate surgery was "genius." The idea of a small incision with the robot was attractive given the nature of the surgery, but there was no evidence that using the robot improved health outcomes.* (See the robotic surgery case study summary.)

Robotic Surgery

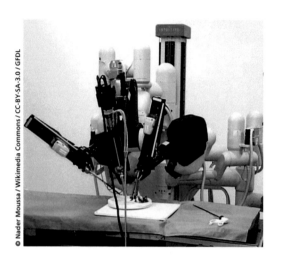

The Technology: Robotically assisted laparoscopic surgery couples the surgeon's movements to those of a remote-controlled robot, thus eliminating tremor. Pioneered in the 1980s, robotically assisted surgery spread widely into surgical procedures in cardiology, cardiothoracic surgery, general surgery, urology, gynecology, pediatrics, vascular surgery, neurosurgery, and orthopedics (Glassman et al., 1992; Camarillo, Krummel, and Salisbury, 2004; Mack, 2001).

Rapid Adoption, Substantial Cost Increase: Over the past five to seven years, robotic technology has been rapidly adopted in both Europe and the United States. In 2010, more than 200,000 robotically assisted procedures were performed (Barbash and Glied, 2010; Zhao and Liu, 2012; Matthews, 2012). But proliferation has come at substantial cost: Overall, robotic assistance increases the cost of a typical surgery by approximately 13 percent. The da Vinci Surgical System, although not the first system introduced, currently dominates the market.

Adoption has been most dramatic in prostatectomy procedures. Although the technology has been available for a little more than a decade, about 80 percent of all radical prostatectomies in the United States today are performed with robotic assistance (Su, 2010). Recent increases in the surgical treatment of prostate cancer appear to be largely driven by acquisition of robotic surgical systems.

Increasingly Profound Effects on Health Care Practice, Training, and Spending: Initially, the primary effect of robots appeared to be attracting surgical volume to the hospitals that acquired them. By 2009, the 35 percent of hospitals that had one or more surgical robots performed 85 percent of all radical prostatectomies (Stitzenberg et al., 2012). Robots also influenced surgical training and practice. By 2010, fully half of practicing urologists reported that they used the robotic technique in either all or some of their cases. Despite claims that the minimally invasive technique reduces blood loss and speeds recovery, there is worrisome evidence that men undergoing robot-assisted prostatectomy are less likely to undergo pelvic lymph node dissection (Feifer et al., 2011), an important procedure to check for cancer spread. Moreover, use of robotic technology is growing rapidly among patients who are far less likely to benefit from the technology and may even be harmed. This includes men with low-risk prostate cancer and medically fragile and elderly men at high risk of noncancer mortality.

The Available Science Does Not Support Proliferation: Despite widespread adoption in the United States, there is no good evidence that robotically assisted radical prostatectomies produce better outcomes or reduce serious side effects relative to manual radical prostatectomy. Use of the robotic approach has been associated with shorter lengths of stay, lower rates of blood transfusion, and lower postoperative respiratory complications (Hu et al., 2009). However, the robotic approach is also associated with more frequent surgical complications, including urinary incontinence, genitourinary complications, and erectile dysfunction.

A Medical "Arms Race": The evidence to date suggests that hospitals and health care systems are primarily acquiring robotic technology to compete for market share. This has increased costs by triggering a dramatic increase in the number of radical surgical prostate extirpations performed annually in the United States without evidence that these extra surgeries are helping patients more than less costly alternatives, such as conventional therapy, radiation treatment, or "watchful waiting."

Another example is proton beam radiation therapy (PBRT), a high-tech alternative to conventional radiation therapy. PBRT requires an enormous and costly facility (approximately $220 million) and is substantially more expensive than more conventional treatments. Because PBRT targets radiation at the location of the cancer, the presumption is that patients suffer fewer side effects. Because some have used this assertion to raise ethical concerns about using randomized controlled trials (RCTs) to assess the health benefits of PBRT, there is virtually no empirical evidence about the health benefits of PBRT.

In 2010, there were seven PBRT centers operating in different parts of the country (*Oncology Times*, 2010, five-part series: Keller, 2010a; Keller, 2010b; Rosenthal, 2010a; Rosenthal, 2010b; and Rosenthal, 2010c). As of October 2013, there were 11 centers operating in the United States and another 13 being developed (National Association for Proton Therapy, 2013). Competing health systems in Washington, D.C., recently announced that each is building its own facility. A prominent oncologist has commented, "We don't have the evidence that there's a need for [proton beam facilities] in terms of medical care. They're simply done to generate profits" (Gold, 2013).

What Drives the Medical Arms Race?

Despite some improvements in payment policy—such as prospective payment systems—hospitals, other facilities, and specialized medical groups continue to use high-tech capabilities to attract business. In most cases, the fundamental goal seems to be financial. Many of our interview subjects supported the views that expensive technologies are used as a competitive tool and that financial considerations are a fundamental reason for acquiring them. For example, one of our interview subjects stated that *in our system there's an intrinsic tension between containing costs and open competition between hospitals—they're competing on recruitment of patients and volume* [DEV3]. Another interview subject [PROV1] reported that *a key avenue for attracting more business is offering capabilities that suit the preferences of leading local physicians, many of whom want to use the latest technologies, especially if doing so is relatively lucrative.* As noted by one provider we interviewed [PROV6], *there's no question that hospitals use technology to market their services.* For products that increase spending without commensurate improvements in medical outcomes, the extent of this form of competition in a local health care market depends on how many hospitals and physicians are at financial risk for providing associated services. As previously discussed, providers are increasingly being put at financial risk, and this trend is likely to continue.

The Medical Arms Race Can Substantially Affect Incentives of Inventors

Hospitals, other facilities, and physician groups purchase expensive medical equipment anticipating that they will recoup the purchase price through payments for using the equipment to treat or diagnose patients. If a provider who owns the equipment cannot keep it operating at or near full capacity for patients for whom it promises large health benefits, financial incentives encourage providers to use the equipment for patients for whom the health benefits—but not the associated spending—is much lower. An example of this is leasing MRI machines to orthopedic surgeons. The extent of such behavior and its effects on spending and health are unknown.

One interviewee [GENX6] highlighted the implications for invention: *Inventors won't be steered toward high-value innovation when we continue to reward low-value innovation. If the marketplace rewards the use of minimally useful imaging devices on a volume basis, the innovation process is distorted.* This aspect of the medical arms race may also be viewed as a form of treatment creep. Most importantly for our analysis, low-value utilization associated with the medical arms race often offers large financial rewards for inventors and their investors. As a result, products that are likely to trigger medical arms races become more attractive to inventors and investors, and products that would offer greater value to society become relatively unattractive.

CHAPTER FIVE

Policy Options to Improve the U.S. Medical Product Innovation System

We have described how several features of the U.S. health care environment create socially undesirable financial incentives for medical product inventors and investors. Our policy goals would be advanced by altering these incentives. The literature, our interviews, our case studies, and discussions with other experts suggest that the decisions of health care inventors and investors are strongly influenced by (1) the costs and risks of product invention, (2) the costs and risks of FDA review ("approval"), and (3) market rewards and risks ("adoption"). Policy options can change the relative costs, rewards, and risks at one or more stages of the innovation pathway.

In this chapter, we describe ten policy options pertaining to drugs and devices that might decrease spending with little sacrifice in health, enhance the prospects that new products are worth the extra spending, or accomplish both. To develop these policy options, we first considered (1) costs and risks along the innovation pathway, (2) policy suggestions contained in the literature, and (3) ideas from technical expert panel members and interviewees. We then brainstormed about the kinds of changes in public and private policy that could substantially ameliorate problems associated with our five themes (lack of basic scientific knowledge, costs and risks of FDA approval, inadequate rewards for medical products that could decrease spending, treatment creep, and the medical arms race). The ten options we present are the ones that we think are most promising based on all of our sources of information and our judgment about which of the many options we considered are most likely to have major impact.

None of our policy options is detailed enough to be implemented. Fleshing out their details would take substantial effort and might require trial and error, particularly if the policies are novel. However, a current lack of specific, implementable approaches is not sufficient reason to dismiss an option. The United States spends trillions of dollars annually on health care; thus, the potential benefits of defining and implementing well-designed versions of any of the options we suggest could dwarf the costs of doing so.

The options could be implemented singly or in various combinations. Moreover, the effects of implementing any of them will likely depend on how other options are focused and implemented. For example, policies could be focused on curing or preventing particular medical conditions that involve high current and future spending, such as Alzheimer's disease, diabetes, or heart failure. They could also be directed at precursors to expensive chronic diseases, such as obesity or hypertension. Preventive interventions may, however, increase or decrease spending (Cohen, Neumann, and Weinstein, 2008; Russell, 2009).

Changing the decisions of inventors and investors requires changing their financial incentives, which are shaped by the costs and risks associated with the invention process and FDA approval processes, as well as the market rewards and risks associated with adoption (Figure 5.1). Inventors and investors might be willing to incur costs and accept risks if the prospect for market rewards is strong. There are also market risks, however, such as the possibilities that a competitor will introduce a superior product or the payment environment will change in ways that make the product less profitable.

Some policy options would affect inventor and investor decisions without changing the market environment; others would operate through market changes. Policies with *direct* effects on inventor and investor incentives—and thereby their decisions— lower invention or approval costs and risks. Policies with *indirect* effects change incentives of inventors and investors by altering the market rewards and risks of an invention effort under consideration.

Policies with direct effects have the advantage of potentially affecting product invention decisions sooner than policies with indirect effects. For example, to indirectly alter an inventor's behavior, policies must alter not only markets for medical products; inventors and investors must understand that the market environment has changed and expect those changes to persist. Major changes in the market environment can take years to play out. The impact of these changes on inventor and investor decisions would then take several more years.

However, policies with direct effects have two disadvantages. First, options with indirect effects can decrease spending faster. This is because changes in payer, provider, and patient incentives could change their patterns of product utilization—and begin to reduce spending—fairly quickly. In contrast, while direct policies will change invention incentives almost immediately, changes in what medical products are available in the United States would take several more years. Second, many policy options

Figure 5.1
Costs, Rewards, and Risks in Invention Decisions

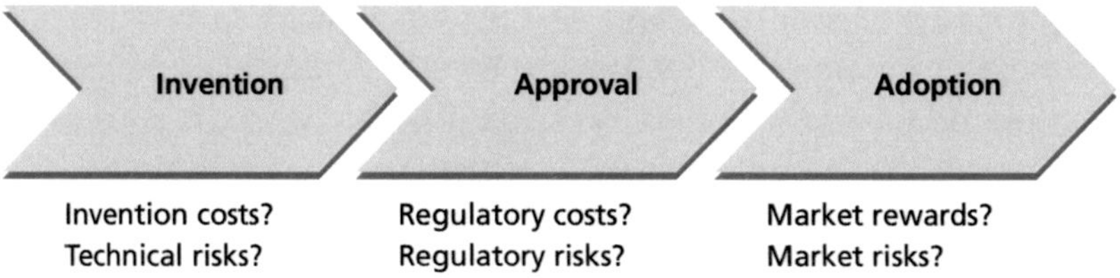

Invention	Approval	Adoption
Invention costs? Technical risks?	Regulatory costs? Regulatory risks?	Market rewards? Market risks?

RAND RR308-5.1

to directly alter inventive activity seem to require implementation on a product-by-product basis. In contrast, some policies that could alter inventive behavior indirectly by reshaping markets for medical products would influence incentives for invention for all or broad classes of medical products (e.g., pharmaceuticals, implanted devices, expensive medical equipment, EHRs).

It is difficult to predict whether a particular policy option would be more likely to help reduce spending (our first policy goal) or to increase spending while also providing commensurate health benefits (our second policy goal). Ultimately, the actual effects of policy changes associated with any option will depend on details of policy design and implementation.

Options to Reduce Costs and Risks of Invention and Approval

We present five options for encouraging the invention of drugs and devices that would further our policy goals directly by reducing costs and/or risks at the invention and approval stages:

1. Enable more creativity in funding basic science.
2. Offer prizes for inventions.
3. Buy out patents.
4. Establish a public-interest investment fund.
5. Expedite FDA reviews and approvals.

Enable More Creativity in Funding Basic Science

Invention of new medical technologies typically builds on a base of basic biomedical science, and a lack of adequate scientific knowledge impedes invention and pursuit of FDA approval. This policy option addresses our theme about the lack of basic scientific knowledge. It is not, however, a proposal for more NIH funding of basic research; rather, it would call on NIH to use its scarce funds to promote additional creativity in the basic scientific work that it funds.

NIH, the largest funder of biomedical research in the world, spent almost $31 billion in fiscal year 2012 on medical research (NIH, 2012). Major breakthroughs in medical product invention—only some of which can be expected to reduce spending—often require earlier breakthroughs in basic science, which likely require many scientists to pursue innovative and risky research programs. As part of the NIH Common Fund, for example, which was created by Congress in 2006, NIH dedicated about $123 million (roughly 0.4 percent of NIH's total research spending) to "high-risk, high-reward" research in 2013 (NIH, 2013a, 2013b). This development, modest as it is, seems to be a step in the right direction and might best be expanded.

By and large, however, NIH still relies on traditional criteria for choosing what research proposals to fund, an approach that avoids risks and is intolerant of failure (Fang and Casadevall, 2009). A potential model for NIH—or another HHS agency willing to support higher-risk scientific endeavors—is the Howard Hughes Medical Institute (HHMI). HHMI provides about $700 million annually to fund academic scientists. It funds scientists rather than projects, encourages risk-taking, and seems more willing than NIH is to provide additional funding to scientists whose past risky endeavors did not pan out (HHMI, 2013; Azoulay, Graff Zivin, and Manso, 2011). (The Advanced Research Projects Agency—Energy [ARPA-E], which is focused on clean energy, is another such model.) There is some empirical evidence that, other things being equal, scientists funded by HHMI are responsible for "higher levels of breakthrough innovation" than NIH-funded scientists (Azoulay, Graff Zivin, and Manso, 2011, p. 550).

By their very nature, the outcomes of basic scientific activities are unpredictable. Presumably, then, some new medical technologies made possible by higher-risk and higher-return biomedical research would decrease spending, and others would increase it.

Offer Prizes for Inventions

One way to increase efforts to invent new products is to offer a "prize" to the first individual or group that invents a drug or device meeting specific criteria. Such prizes would be offered before a qualifying product has been invented. This policy option responds to our theme about inadequate rewards for inventing products that could lower spending.

It is probably infeasible to offer prizes large enough on their own to motivate drug inventors and investors to embark on a product invention effort; however, the invention costs of some devices might be small enough for the prospect of a prize to suffice. Prizes—even when discounted to account for the probability of winning—could induce product invention efforts that are not far from being funded in the absence of a potential prize.

The best strategy might be to offer large numbers of fairly small prizes in the hope of making failures small and successes big. Whatever form prizes take, their availability should be widely publicized to disciplines outside health-related ones: Prizes have often been won by inventors who lacked expertise in the fields regarded as most closely related to the problem (Lakhani et al., 2006; Lakhani and Jeppesen, 2007).

Prizes might be offered by such public entities as CMS, private health care systems seeking to reduce their costs, philanthropists and charitable foundations, or public-private partnerships. Prizes for invention have a long history in other contexts (Brennan, Maccauley, and Whitefoot, 2012; Rosenberg, 2012), and there is an extensive literature about them (Knowledge Ecology International, undated). Some organizations—such as the X Prize Foundation and InnoCentive—offer prizes in a variety of technological areas, while others focus on medicine and health care. (See Knowledge Ecology International [2008] for many examples.) Many health-related prizes aim to spur development of drugs to address "neglected" diseases that are particularly important in low-income countries (Glennerster and Kremer, 2000; Stiglitz and Jayadev, 2010).

Most often, prizes have been cash payments awarded when the competition's criteria are met. However, a prize could also be paid later as, for example, shares of savings to the Medicare program that could be attributed to the invention. Because Medicare spent roughly $536 billion in 2012 (Kaiser Family Foundation, 2012), even a small share of Medicare savings could amount to hundreds of millions or even billions of dollars. New federal legislation would be required to enable CMS to offer prizes.

Buy Out Selected Patents

Purchasing patents on products that have already been invented is another way to increase rewards for inventing products that are unattractive to inventors and investors. (If offers to buy patents—including specified criteria and attractive purchase prices— were made prior to invention, patent buyouts would work similarly to prizes.) Patents could be purchased by public agencies, private philanthropic entities, or public-private partnerships. We anticipate that—because of budget constraints, for example—a fairly small number of patents could be purchased and that patent purchasers would need to be very selective.

The purpose of post-invention patent buyouts would be to ensure that a product that would reduce spending is commercialized and offered at low prices, thus encouraging wider use. Thus, this policy option addresses our theme about inadequate rewards for inventing products that could lower spending, particularly the limited rewards for product manufacturers to compete on price. As discussed in the context of that theme, we would expect some increase in utilization to result from lower prices because some patients are price sensitive (such as uninsured patients and insured patients who have not exceeded their deductibles or who face relatively high levels of cost-sharing). Low prices could be achieved in different ways. For example, the purchaser could put the patent in the public domain, where broad use could generate competition, or the patent could be licensed to one or multiple entities, specifying the amount they could charge for the product. It is possible that lower prices per episode of care would expand utilization so much that total spending would increase.

Determining a purchase price is a major implementation issue for patent buyouts. At least two different approaches have been explored. Guell and Fischbaum (1995) focus on pharmaceuticals and suggest that purchase prices should approximate "the expected net present value of future monopoly profits" (p. 214). Kremer (1998) noted several problems with administratively determined purchase prices and proposed using an auction mechanism.

The amount of money required to purchase the patent for a high-impact product that could decrease spending might be very considerable, and more so if other policy measures are implemented that would increase demand for such products. When this is the case, instead of buying out patents with cash, the best approach might be to offer (as we discussed in the context of prizes) the patent owner a share of Medicare savings attributable to the product.

Establish a Public-Interest Investment Fund

Even if a motivated team of inventors has a promising idea for a product that could decrease spending, they might not be able to attract sufficient funds from private investors to support invention. This is because—as emphasized in our theme about inadequate rewards for inventing products that could lower spending—market rewards for inventing products that could decrease spending are often too low to be attractive to private investors.

A public-interest investment fund (PIIF) could finance invention efforts (including clinical trials) that are not attractive to private investors under current institutional arrangements. Financing could also be coupled with additional incentives—for example, lump sum or gain-sharing prizes or patent purchases—to motivate inventors to work hard and smart. A viable PIIF would require ongoing revenue sources, the most promising of which might be shared savings to the Medicare program.

Establishing and operating a PIIF would confront several challenges. First, the fund might require more money to get started than would be needed to offer prizes or buy out patents. In principle, the start-up financing could come from NIH or from CMS if new legislation permitted. Second, making wise investment decisions and managing product invention efforts are challenging tasks even for people with the best expertise and judgment. Relying entirely or primarily on public officials or employees to do so raises the kinds of concerns—which we share—raised in the general debate about technology policy and governments "picking winners." Most of the people who are in the best position to assess the promise of potential new drugs and devices work in the private sector—in venture capital or other private-equity firms, for example.

How could the PIIF make it attractive to such people to participate in choosing projects to fund and managing the associated R&D? A promising approach might be a private-public partnership in which private investors were allowed to invest in projects supported by the PIIF. Payoffs for success would include shared Medicare savings. Moreover, if such a partnership attracted money from private venture capital and equity funds, it could reduce the amount of public money required.

Expedite FDA Reviews and Approvals for Products That Decrease Spending

Even when the FDA does a great job in assuring safety and efficacy, FDA review and approval require product inventors to incur considerable expenditures, add risks, keep money tied up, and delay receipt of revenues from U.S. markets. This policy option would involve speeding up—without weakening—the review and approval process for drugs and devices that could be expected to lead to substantial spending decreases, making investment in such products more attractive. This option follows from our theme about costs and risks involved in gaining FDA approval.

Four mechanisms already exist to speed FDA review and approval for qualifying drugs and devices: the "fast track," "accelerated approval," "priority review," and "break-through therapy" mechanisms. Current eligibility criteria for using these mechanisms focus solely on such health effects as the expectation that a product will fill an unmet need for a serious condition (FDA, 2013a). Most important for present purposes, there is no existing mechanism to expedite FDA reviews for products that appear likely to decrease spending. Creating such a mechanism, which would require new legislation, would expand the FDA's mission beyond safety and efficacy to include spending. (The ACA does, however, provide for tax credits for efforts to invent therapies that, among other things, "show a reasonable potential to . . . . Reduce long-term growth in health care costs in the United States . . . ." [NIH, 2010]).

In implementing this option, policymakers—at the FDA or elsewhere—would need to address questions such as the following: How should it be decided whether a product truly has the potential to decrease spending? Should applicants be required to commit to a price in order to qualify for expedited review? How would the FDA handle a situation in which a product has been modified—e.g., a new dosage or delivery approach for a drug or a modification of a device?

Implementation Challenges

Implementation of these options would require policymakers to confront at least two challenges. First, some options require identification of drugs and devices that would likely decrease spending *before* they are invented (e.g., establishing criteria for awarding prizes or allocating support from the public-interest investment fund prior to product invention). The second challenge is determining, once a product has been invented, whether it will decrease or has decreased spending and, if so, by how much (this information would be needed to buy out patents or determine eligibility for expedited FDA review).

Options to Increase Market Rewards

We now present five options for encouraging the invention and adoption of drugs and devices by increasing market rewards for products that would further our two policy goals and/or decrease market rewards for inventions that would not further our goals:

1. Reform Medicare payment policies.
2. Reform Medicare coverage policies.
3. Coordinate FDA approval and CMS coverage processes.
4. Increase demand for products that decrease spending.
5. Produce more and more-timely technology assessments.

Reform Medicare Payment Policies

This option addresses three of our themes: inadequate rewards for products that could lower spending and undesirable forms of treatment creep and medical arms races. Several ongoing efforts by CMS that will tend to advance our two policy goals are discussed in Chapter Four in the context of inadequate rewards for products that could lower spending.

If CMS were allowed to consider cost in determining payment rates—which would require new legislation—it could set Medicare rates to save money in the short term and increase incentives to invent products that could reduce spending in the longer term. It appears, however, that CMS may be able to pursue pricing reform through its Innovation Center (CMS, undated [a]).

A widely recognized possibility would be for CMS to move more rapidly away from FFS payment to payment approaches that put providers at financial risk for doing more than is needed to provide quality care and/or using unnecessarily expensive interventions. This would increase providers' demand for less costly approaches to care, which could increase demand for medical products with the potential to lower spending. Under revised payment arrangements, inventors who create a treatment that is substantially cheaper but just as effective as an existing technology could expect a large market. Similarly, those who invent an expensive product that provides little health benefit would be less likely to reap large market rewards.

Payment approaches that improve incentives to save money include (1) bundled payment arrangements for episodes of care (Luft, 2009; Pham et al., 2010; Altman, 2012; Emanuel, 2013), already implemented in Medicare prospective payment systems for inpatient and outpatient hospital care; (2) capitated payment arrangements involving fixed payments per person to cover all care, which are already implemented in Medicare Part C and are common in Medicaid; and (3) reference pricing schemes that involve setting payment rates no higher than those currently paid for equally effective products and services (Robinson and MacPherson, 2012). The extent to which putting providers at financial risk—through bundled or capitated payment arrangements, for example—would decrease spending depends in part on how much of any provider savings is passed on to payers and consumers. In principle, this in turn depends on the degrees of price competition among providers and among payers, which differ across local health insurance and health care markets.

Some ACOs under the ACA involve capitated payment and also include shared savings provisions (Berwick, 2011; American Medical Association, 2011). CMS might also consider performance-based payment approaches for products it pays for separately, such as drugs administered in physician offices or medical devices implanted in hospitals. Incentives might include bonuses for especially good health outcomes and penalties for the opposite.

Appropriate Medicare payment rates for technologies and associated services are particularly difficult to determine when a technology is new and there is little, if any, clinical experience with it. A "dynamic pricing" scheme might be used for new products. With dynamic pricing, the initial Medicare payment rate could be set on the basis of an optimistic assessment of the health benefits of a new product but could then be reduced a few years later unless the product is shown to support the initial optimism (Pearson and Bach, 2010; Emanuel and Pearson, 2012).

Reform Medicare Coverage Policies

CMS could also change its coverage determination processes and policies in ways that would increase the health benefits per dollar of Medicare spending. Since many private payers apparently follow Medicare's lead in coverage determinations, the spending effects of such policies could extend to care that is paid for privately.

To further our two policy goals, CMS could expand use of its "coverage with evidence" process by which coverage is provided on the condition that the manufacturer conducts and reports additional research (Tunis and Pearson, 2006; Carnahan, 2007; Daniel, Rubens, and McClellan, 2013; Neumann and Chambers, 2013).

In addition, Congress requires Medicare to pay for a cancer drug for indications that have not been approved by the FDA as long as the drug is listed for that indication in one of several pharmaceutical compendia; listing often occurs despite scant evidence of effectiveness (Tillman et al., 2009; Sox, 2009; Bach, 2009). If new legislation permitted, Medicare could stop covering off-label use of some very expensive cancer and other specialty drugs (Tillman et al., 2009; Bach, 2009). Doing so could reduce the scope of undesirable treatment creep.

Moreover, a substantial, but unknown, proportion of the off-label use of cancer drugs is for terminally ill patients, for whom treatment often greatly reduces quality of life while rarely adding more than a few weeks or months of life (Weeks et al., 2012; Gawande, 2010). It seems likely that many such patients would opt for palliative and hospice care if they were well informed about the benefits, costs, and alternatives to continued efforts to extend their lives. For example, there is some evidence that doctors—who are well informed—opt for palliative and hospice care for themselves at considerably higher rates than do other terminally ill patients (Murray, 2011, 2012). Expanding use of palliative and hospice care might also reduce spending. For example, Medicare spending is about $2,500 to $6,500 less for terminally ill patients who use hospice services (Kelley et al., 2013).

Medicare and private payers could also stop covering medically inappropriate tests and procedures involving expensive drugs and devices. Several possibilities along these lines have been identified by the Choosing Wisely initiative, started by the American Board of Internal Medicine Foundation (ABIM Foundation) and Consumer Reports, in which more than 50 specialty societies participate. Each society has identified diagnostic and therapeutic procedures—some of which involve medical products—that are often unnecessary and may even be harmful (Choosing Wisely, 2014; Cassel and Guest, 2012; Levey, 2013). It is unclear whether new legislation would be required for

CMS to move in this direction. This is because the Choosing Wisely initiative identifies forms of care that specialty societies indicate should not be provided; thus, it may be that most of them do not satisfy Medicare's legislative mandate to cover "reasonable and necessary" care.

In many instances, withdrawing coverage might reduce the prevalence of undesirable forms of treatment creep and decrease the financial benefits to hospitals and other facilities of some forms of the new medical arms race. However, it is not clear that withdrawing coverage would reduce spending. For example, in some instances providers might shift to even more expensive interventions that are covered by Medicare when they cannot be paid for interventions that have lost Medicare coverage.

Coordinate FDA Approval and CMS Coverage Processes

Medicare pays separately for Part B drugs and some medical devices. (Some other drugs and devices are paid for as part of prospective, bundled, or capitated payment schemes, such as Medicare [Part C] Advantage plans.) Another potential way to encourage invention of products that could lower spending is to reduce manufacturers' costs and delays by coordinating the CMS coverage and payment determination processes with the FDA review and approval processes. Coordination might involve, for example, concurrent reviews by the FDA for approval and CMS for coverage, with CMS specifying early on what evidence it requires to secure Medicare coverage in addition to what the FDA requires for approval. To further reduce manufacturers' time costs and risks, CMS might also specify what information would help it determine a payment rate.

This option, which is aimed at increasing the attractiveness of investing in products that could help lower spending—could be viewed as an extension of the FDA's Innovation Pathway 2.0 initiative (FDA, 2012). This initiative engages device innovators earlier in the FDA process (FDA, 2012). The initiative could be expanded to include drugs, CMS could also get involved in the process earlier than usual, and scientists from NIH could be included as members of the "network of experts." The Office of the Secretary of the U.S. Department of Health and Human Services would be an appropriate venue for considering the potential for coordination, the pros and cons of different approaches, and potential new requirements and rules. In fact, the FDA and CMS have a pilot program involving concurrent FDA review and the CMS process for national coverage determinations for some medical devices, and there are other existing forms of FDA-CMS coordination, some of which involve other federal agencies as well (Chambers, 2012; FDA, 2014). Lessons learned from these efforts could be very helpful in fleshing out details for this policy option.

Increase Demand for Products That Could Decrease Spending

One of our themes pertains to inadequate financial rewards for inventing products that could reduce spending. Demand for such products could be increased by changing the financial incentives of providers and patients.

Such payment approaches as bundled or capitated payment could reduce provider rewards for low-value care. Incentives for providers to provide low-cost care could be fortified through gain-sharing arrangements. For example, hospitals subject to pro-spective payment approaches could share some of their cost savings with physicians (Ketchum and Furukawa, 2008).

Increased cost-sharing could give patients incentives to request lower-cost services or reject physician recommendations for high-cost ones. Expanding use of HDHPs could have similar effects (Lo Sasso, Helmchen, and Kaestner, 2010; Buntin et al., 2011; Haviland et al., 2011). Increased use of HDHPs might increase substantially under the ACA in the small-employer market (Wharam, Ross-Degnan, and Rosenthal, 2013) but may decline substantially in the individual market (Andrews, 2013).

We do not think, however, that increasing cost-sharing across the board would be desirable. Besides making high-value care unaffordable for some Americans and decreasing the benefits of financial risk-sharing within insurance pools, across-the-board increases in cost-sharing or wider use of HDHPs would lead patients to cut back on both low- and high-value care (Baicker and Goldman, 2011; Chandra, Cutler, and Song, 2012). In short, increasing cost-sharing across the board is a very blunt instrument.

A considerably more promising alternative is expanding the use of value-based insurance designs (VBIDs; Chernew, Rosen, and Fendrick, 2007; Fendrick, Chernew, and Levi, 2009; Chernew et al., 2010; Fendrick, Smith, and Chernew, 2010; Robinson, 2010; University of Michigan Center for Value-Based Insurance Design, 2012, 2013). This is because VBIDs can address spending in ways that are much more likely to increase value. The VBID model is driven by the concept of *clinical nuance*, which rec-ognizes that (1) medical services differ in the benefits they provide; and (2) the health benefit derived from a specific service depends on what patient uses it, as well as when and where the service is provided. VBIDs improve the incentives of both consumers and product inventors by setting cost-sharing rates so that low-value services become more costly to patients than high-value ones, thus decreasing utilization of the former relative to the latter. However, improving incentives in this way is easier said than done: A service can be high-value for some patients and low-value, or even harmful, for others, and for many services there is a lot of uncertainty about which patients fall into which category. The desirability of designing insurance schemes that incorporate clinical nuance leads to our final policy option.

Produce More and More-Timely Technology Assessments

Poor understanding of the safety and effectiveness of many medical technologies can fuel undesirable medical arms races and contribute to undesirable treatment creep. Lack of knowledge is also a major impediment to implementing VBIDs. Health technology assessments (HTAs)—comparative effectiveness and cost-effectiveness analyses, for example—provide systematic evidence about the safety, efficacy, effectiveness, and cost of drugs, devices, and procedures. Such evidence can help payers and providers decide whether, when, and for whom it is more or less wise to use a particular technology. Moreover, one of the major barriers to adoption of telemedicine is the lack of good evidence about its costs and health effects. (See the telemedicine case study summary.)

Telemedicine

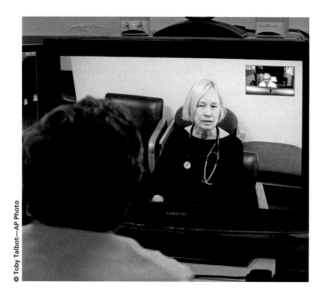

© Toby Talbot—AP Photo

The Technology: Telemedicine is the delivery of health care services across a geographical distance using communications technology. Its primary goal is to extend the reach of generalist and specialist health care providers to geographically remote or underserved areas and to serve homebound or isolated patients who have limited ability to travel.

Development: Telegraphy, the original form of telemedicine, was used to facilitate medical communication during the Civil War. Technical advances, such as closed circuit television and satellite communications, in the 1960s to 1980s laid the conceptual foundations for modern telemedicine. Federal agencies, including the National Aeronautics and Space Administration; the U.S. Department of Health, Education, and Welfare; and the U.S. National Science Foundation were major facilitators. However, demonstration projects could not be sustained when public funding expired because there was no way to reimburse the service.

Federal agencies and the U.S. Army played important roles in the 1990s and 2000s, exploiting new technological developments, including the rise of the Internet. Advances in technology spurred incorporation of telemedicine into clinical practice and expansion into academic environments. Real-time telemedicine applications, such as telepsychiatry, emerged as an alternative to face-to-face treatment.

Technological Barriers to Adoption Have Fallen: Rapid advances in telecommunications and computer technology over the last ten to 20 years, especially the switch to digital technology and the decreasing cost of information transmission, have helped to promote expansion of telemedicine. The Internet, computer networks, and web-based applications have enabled real-time telemedicine applications that would have been technically impossible a generation ago.

Major Barriers to Widespread Adoption Remain: The most formidable barrier to widespread adoption of telemedicine is the current system of medical licensure regulation. All state medical licensing boards require a physician engaging in telemedicine to hold a medical license in the state where the patient is located. There is no reciprocity between states to allow a physician licensed in one state to practice telemedicine medicine in another, despite the existence of national board examinations, national specialty certification, and similar medical licensing requirements between the states. As a result, few physicians are legally credentialed to provide telemedical care across state lines to patients in remote or underserved areas.

Other impediments to adoption include financial barriers (high technology costs, insufficient Medicare reimbursement for telemedicine services, state and private-sector restrictions on coverage), provider reluctance to invest time and resources in learning new technology, and medico-legal concerns.

Evidence of Effectiveness Lacking: Telemedicine's impact on costs and quality of care has not been convincingly demonstrated. However, most of the studies conducted to date have compared telemedicine versus face-to-face health care by a licensed health care provider or expert consultant, rather than telemedicine versus no provider (the true alternative in many rural areas). Without adequate large-scale evaluations, it is difficult to demonstrate telemedicine's potential impact. Prospective research on its impact in austere settings that currently have inadequate access to care could fill a major gap in the telemedicine literature and, depending on the findings, encourage greater stakeholder support.

"Adoption Block": Telemedicine is an example of adoption block: The technology is feasible and highly promising, but it cannot gain market traction because its adoption threatens the interests of powerful institutions and groups, such as local health care practitioners and state licensing boards. Where parochial concerns do not exist and reimbursement is assured—for instance, teleradiology—telemedicine has flourished.

Telemedicine has the potential to increase provider efficiency, promote health care equity, and enhance access to care in geographically remote and underserved communities. But until sufficient will is mustered to break down the political and regulatory barriers impeding its adoption, its promise will be largely unfulfilled.

HTAs are conducted by public entities, such as NIH, the Agency for Health Care Research and Quality, and CMS (which conducts HTAs as part of Medicare's process for making National Coverage Determinations), as well as the VA. HTAs are also conducted by private organizations. Some of them—such as the Blue Cross and Blue Shield Association Technology Evaluation Center and the Institute for Clinical and Economic Review—share their assessments without payment; others—such as Hayes, Inc., and the ECRI Institute—do not (Harrington, 2011). The comparative effectiveness studies being sponsored by PCORI should also be helpful in this regard. Production of HTAs might also be facilitated by conducting head-to-head ("equivalence") clinical trials of new drugs or devices versus older products in widespread use, perhaps as part of a new FDA mandate to require such trials for approval.

Unfortunately, it can take years to perform high-quality HTAs. Often by the time an HTA is completed, the technology has evolved (e.g., there is a newer, improved version) or new alternatives have emerged (e.g., an even newer drug or device has been introduced). As Newhouse (2002, p. 18) put it: "rapid change makes knowledge quickly obsolete and places a heavy burden on mechanisms that enable physicians and other health professionals to keep up."

We will learn more about the comparative effectiveness of many medical interventions in the coming years through research supported by PCORI. A provision of the ACA, however, greatly limits consideration of costs in research supported by PCORI (A. Garber and Sox, 2010).

An emerging private-sector model for producing timely HTAs could be encouraged by public policy and/or imitated by entities that produce or fund HTAs. Specifically, rather than spending years to produce an HTA, and updating it years later if at all, a commercial entity called UpToDate appears to keep abreast of new evidence by fairly frequent literature searches and revises its HTAs whenever new findings warrant (UpToDate, 2014). There appears to be no publicly available information on which to judge whether this model is likely to address large numbers of technologies or to help with the timeliness problem for the technologies that are assessed. For example, we cannot tell how frequently UpToDate reviews literature and revises its HTAs, how many subscribers it has or the rate of growth of the subscriber base, whether it has commercial competitors, and so on. But given the value of HTAs, this model is worth serious exploration.

Summary

Several well-known features of the U.S. health care environment, characterized by our study themes, create financial incentives that reward inventors and private investors for inventing and marketing products that tend to increase health care spending, whether or not they also substantially improve health. Moreover, inventors appear to have relatively weak incentives to create products that could decrease spending.

The policy options presented in this chapter, summarized in Figure 5.2, are intended to realign the incentives of inventors and investors. In the aggregate, they could redirect inventive effort toward products with the potential to further our policy goals.

Figure 5.2
Summary of Policy Options for Redirecting Inventive Efforts

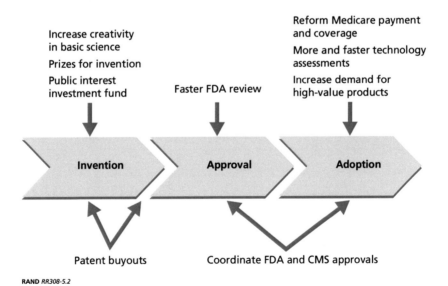

CHAPTER SIX

In Conclusion

The rate of growth of U.S. spending on health care seems to have declined in recent years, and some ongoing trends will help reduce spending. The facts remain, however, that spending on health care in the United States constrains our opportunities to further major public and private priorities other than health, and there is substantial room for reducing spending in ways requiring only fairly small sacrifices in population health.

Many have pointed to new medical technologies, including new drugs and devices, as a leading source of high levels and growth rates of spending on health care. Previous studies have explored ways to rein in spending, but not ways to change which new medical products are invented and marketed in the United States. Thus, our analysis is novel in that it focuses on the latter.

What can we do to improve matters related to invention? We argue that perverse financial incentives of inventors, investors, payers, providers, and patients are the root cause of the problem. Accordingly, the best hope for fixing the system is to change incentives to further our two policy goals:

1. Reduce total health care spending with the smallest possible loss of health benefits.
2. Ensure that new medical products that increase spending are accompanied by health benefits that are worth the spending increases.

Our analysis of the information we collected and created for this project led us to ten policy options that appear promising for advancing one or both of these goals.

The first five options would decrease costs and risks of inventing new products or obtaining regulatory approval for products that would advance our two policy goals. These options are

1. enabling more creativity in funding basic science
2. offering prizes for inventions
3. buying out patents
4. establishing a public interest investment fund
5. expediting FDA review.

The last five options would increase the market rewards for inventing products that would advance our two policy goals. These options are

1. reforming Medicare payment policies
2. reforming Medicare coverage policies
3. coordinating FDA approval and CMS coverage processes
4. increasing demand for products that decrease spending
5. producing more and more-timely technology assessments.

Several of the options appear to be novel in the context of our two policy goals. Because they are novel, however, there are few precedents or existing analyses to help policymakers design and successfully implement them. In view of how much we spend on health care, the potential benefits of investing in designing and effectively implementing specific policies could well dwarf the costs of doing so. The potential savings to the Medicare program that could result from implementing several of our options represent large pools of money that could be used to supplement financial incentives that would otherwise not suffice to spur invention of drugs and devices that could help advance our two policy goals.

It is important for policymakers to recognize—and take into account—that the costs and benefits of any option will depend on what other policy changes are instituted. For example, the increased use of bundled, capitated, or other payment approaches that increase the financial risk of providers would tend to increase demand and market rewards for products that are likely to reduce spending. In turn, increased demand for such products would tend to (1) increase the value of patents on products that would help lower spending, thus increasing prices required to purchase them, but (2) might have at most minor effects on how much money would be needed to launch and sustain a PIIF.

The stakes in reining in health care spending and getting more health benefits from the money we do spend are so high that we believe all promising options should be considered—*and the sooner the better*. However, as helpful as it may be to change the nature of future drugs and devices, we cannot reasonably expect our two policy goals to be adequately addressed only by changing the incentives of inventors. First, crafting effective policies to influence invention directly will often require policymakers to target particular diseases (such as Alzheimer's disease and diabetes) or disease precursors (such as obesity and hypertension) rather than medical product invention broadly. Second, much of low-value health care spending is not directly related to drugs or devices, and failing to address such spending would indefinitely leave in place some of the causes of low-value spending and utilization.

Multiple stakeholders—including drug and device companies, investors, physicians, hospitals, and others—can be expected to resist many of the policy options we have presented. Fundamentally reforming Medicare would likely meet the most powerful resistance. Nonetheless, we present options to change both Medicare coverage policy and Medicare payment policy. It is hard to be sanguine about moving the needles on spending and value without fundamentally reforming Medicare, which accounts for nearly 20 percent of all U.S. health care spending. The reforms we describe would require new legislation to allow Medicare to explicitly consider costs. We recognize that allowing CMS to consider cost in formulating Medicare payment and coverage policies will be extremely challenging.

Much of the resistance to our policy options may decry "rationing," may be framed in terms of fairness, and may invoke "rights" of access to health care. Indeed, if the policy options we have highlighted were fleshed out and implemented, some U.S. residents would lose medical care that would benefit them. However, because it is often the case that others are paying the bills, it might be appropriate to conceive of "rights" of consumers as pertaining not to all desired health care—effective or not, shockingly expensive or not—but rather as rights only to effective and high-value care.

The longer we wait to institute fundamental reforms, the more money we will spend on health care yielding little or no health benefit—and the harder it will be to achieve other major social priorities.

Cost-Effectiveness and Value

To understand the interaction between innovation and health care spending, we need to understand the circumstances in which medical technology produces better value in health (Sorenson, Drummond, and Khan, 2013). Two main ways of analyzing a policy change such as the introduction of a new product are cost-benefit analysis and cost-effectiveness analysis. Cost-benefit analysis assesses whether a change is worthwhile by valuing the societal costs of the policy by the opportunities forgone to implement it, and valuing the beneficial effects by what the recipients (and others who care about them) would be willing to pay for them. Any policy whose benefits exceed the costs is preferable to the status quo, and the policy with the largest net benefits is best.

Cost-effectiveness analysis is used to solve a different problem. It can help a health agency with a budget get maximum health gains for that budget. A major difference from cost-benefit analysis (and standard welfare economics) is that the agency counts the health gains of rich and poor people in the same way, rather than valuing benefits in terms of individual recipients' willingness to pay. In the private market for health, wealthy people can buy more health, just as they can afford new luxury cars that are safer than old compact vehicles. Nevertheless, for governments or societies with a given health budget, health maximization is a reasonable goal, which reflects desires for justice and taxpayer altruism toward the economically disadvantaged, especially poor children.

Value is defined in terms of cost-effectiveness. The fundamental tool used by cost-effectiveness analysis to maximize population health gains is the incremental cost-effectiveness ratio (ICER). For a new technology, the ICER is the resulting change in costs from the status quo divided by the change in health. It measures how much each additional unit of health costs. In the health-maximizing allocation subject to a constraint on total costs, under certain assumptions, all services that produce health that fall below an ICER threshold are funded, and all services with ICERs above that threshold are not funded. Starting from the services with the lowest ICERs, society funds services up the line until the budget runs out. The ICER when the money runs out is the threshold.

In the real world, there will be many exceptions to this rule, for political, cultural, and ethical reasons. Still, we can use this fundamental concept of cost-effectiveness to define what we mean by high and low value.

Three Types of High-Value Technologies

A new medical technology has both cost and health implications, as illustrated in Figure A.1. Technologies are located in the figure based on their expected lifetime costs and health effects relative to the status quo. So the origin, where the axes cross, represents the status quo. Some new technologies improve health (any point in the top two quadrants of the graph) and others worsen it (any point in the bottom two quadrants). Similarly, some technologies offer cost savings (the left two quadrants), while others lead to higher costs (the right two quadrants). We prefer technologies to the northwest of other technologies, as shown by the arrows, because such technologies provide higher health benefits and lower costs. A new technology can provide positive value by providing greater health benefits, reducing costs, or achieving both.

Technologies like D that fall in the southeast quadrant have higher cost and worse health implications than the status quo—they decrease value and should not be invented or developed. Technologies like A that fall in the northwest quadrant provide

Figure A.1
Cost and Health Quadrants

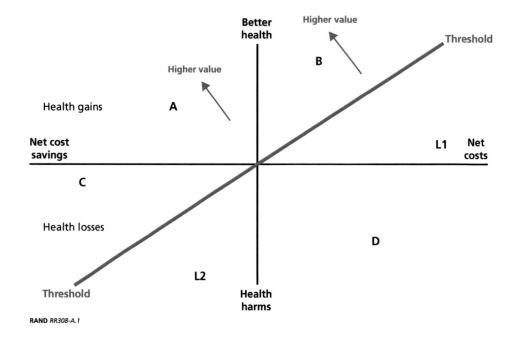

better health at lower cost—clearly they are high-value and worth inventing and using (for the right patients). For technologies like B and C in the other quadrants, there is a trade-off between cost and health benefits—i.e., relative to the status quo, they improve one outcome but worsen the other.

Most of the literature on cost-effectiveness focuses on the northeast quadrant, where technologies are said to be cost-effective or high value if they buy a lot of health per dollar, as B does. In the figure, the cost-effectiveness threshold is represented by a line passing through the origin, whose equation is *Health Gains = ICER × Costs*.

Technologies represented by points such as C, which save a lot of money while sacrificing a little health, are also above the line. In principle, one could take the money saved by C and put it in another service above the threshold, ending up with more health for the same budget, or the savings could be used for some other desirable social goal, such as education, infrastructure, or national defense. So A, B and C all represent desirable, high-value technologies, but L1, L2, and D represent low-value ones. Points such as C often come from stopping something wasteful, such as using a technology represented by the (antipodal) point L1. The people who had benefited from receiving the latter technology may not be happy with this change. In the context of innovation, not inventing L1 would have the benefit C.

An Economic Model of Innovation

A commercial investment to invent a new product is financially worthwhile if the expected discounted downstream profits (or market rewards) outweigh the expected costs of invention and regulatory approval (Goldman and Lakdawalla, 2012). However, an idea may not succeed because of scientific and other uncertainties in invention or approval. Therefore, to calculate expected profits, the potential downstream profits must be multiplied by the probability of successfully getting the product to market. If the costs of invention can be reduced, investments with smaller expected profits become attractive. Investment in inventing technology that decreases spending is often limited by problems in generating downstream profits.

According to standard economic theory, the social value in the United States of a new technology is the marginal utility to U.S. patients (i.e., their willingness to pay for it) minus the extra cost over the lifetime of the technology. (If the technology decreases costs, this value becomes the changes in utility to the patients plus the costs averted.) This value is shared among inventors, payers, providers, and patients. Incentives to invent increase as the share that goes to the inventor rises. Thus, policies that increase that share, such as patent protection, have been used to promote invention. In the limit, inventors get it all, which can be economically efficient, but no one other than inventors (and their investors) benefits from the invention.

After a small-molecule drug has been approved and adopted, its marginal costs of production are usually low enough to be effectively negligible. (Production costs are usually substantial for biologics or large-molecule drugs.) When marginal production costs are very low, almost all revenues are profits, and firms will try to maximize revenues, which are the product of price and volume. If the firm has a patent on a drug that is the only way to treat a class of patients, it can command a high price for it. Me-too drugs—especially generics—will damage the patent holder's bargaining position and force it to lower the price. In markets where a drug has to meet some cost-effectiveness standard, which is not uncommon outside the United States, the price cannot exceed its marginal health value, but this may still be well above the costs of production. In any event, the firm will benefit from increasing volume as long as price exceeds marginal production cost. If neither patients nor providers are greatly concerned with costs, firms may create demand for drugs that do slightly more for health than current ones by various marketing strategies.

When the marginal health benefits exceed the change in out-of-pocket costs, and providers do not care about costs, a drug can be sold widely. For example, treatable illness categories can be expanded. People with prehypertension or prediabetes benefit less from drugs than people with hypertension and diabetes, but their benefit may still exceed their out-of-pocket costs. Over the lifetime of a product, there may also be increased use that is socially desirable because of discovery of different types of patients that benefit or, with practice, improvements that either improve effectiveness or reduce costs.

The cost-effectiveness of any service depends on who gets it. For example, insulin offers high value to people who have diabetes but provides no value and may harm those who do not have diabetes. So a new technology is not represented by a single point in the cost-effects graph (Figure A.1 in Appendix A), but by a different point for each class of patients to which it is applied. For any given cost-effectiveness threshold, we could take all patients whose costs and effects are above the threshold and assume that they and only they will use it. The resulting sum of costs and health benefits represents the optimal use of that technology from the viewpoint of cost-effectiveness. Instead of that ideal, we should calculate costs and effects based on expected or actual use to judge value, just as investors and innovators will use expected profits rather than best-case scenarios to make their decisions.

References

Aaron HJ, "How Not to Reform Medicare," *New England Journal of Medicine*, Vol. 364, No. 17, April 28, 2011, pp. 1588–1589.

Aaron HJ and Reischauer RD, "The Medicare Reform Debate: What Is the Next Step?" *Health Affairs*, Vol. 14, No. 5, 1995, pp. 8–30.

Ackerly DC, Valverde AM, Diener LW, Dossary KL, and Schulman KA, "Fueling Innovation in Medical Devices (and Beyond): Venture Capital in Health Care," *Health Affairs*, web exclusive, December 2, 2008, pp. w68–w75.

AHIP Coverage, "New Report: Medigap Enrollment Continues to Increase," Washington, D.C., May 20, 2013. As of March 15, 2014:
http://www.ahipcoverage.com/2013/05/20/new-report-medigap-enrollment-continues-to-increase/

Altman SH, "The Lessons of Medicare's Prospective Payment System Show That the Bundled Payment Program Faces Challenges," *Health Affairs*, Vol. 31, No. 9, 2012, pp. 1923–1930.

American Medical Association, "Medicare Shared Savings Program: Accountable Care Organizations Final Rule," November 2011. As of January 1, 2014:
http://www.ama-assn.org/resources/doc/washington/medicare-shared-savings-chart.pdf

Andrews M, "Low-Premium, High-Deductible Health Plans Are Endangered by the Affordable Care Act," *Washington Post*, August 12, 2013. As of January 1, 2014:
http://www.washingtonpost.com/national/health-science/
low-premium-high-deductible-health-plans-are-endangered-by-affordable-care-act/
2013/08/12/6b63ffac-fa46-11e2-9bde-7ddaa186b751_print.html

Auerbach DI and Kellermann AL, "A Decade of Health Care Cost Growth Has Wiped Out Real Income Gains for an Average US Family," *Health Affairs*, Vol. 30, No. 9, September 2011, pp. 1620–1636.

Azoulay P, Graff Zivin JS, and Manso G, "Incentives and Creativity: Evidence from the Academic Life Sciences," *RAND Journal of Economics*, Vol. 42, No. 3, 2011, pp. 527–554.

Bach PB, "Limits on Medicare's Ability to Control Rising Spending on Cancer Drugs," *New England Journal of Medicine*, Vol. 360, February 5, 2009, pp. 626–633.

Baciu, Alina, Kathleen Stratton, and Sheila P. Burke, eds., *The Future of Drug Safety: Promoting and Protecting the Health of the Public*, Institute of Medicine of the National Academies, Washington, D.C.: National Academies Press, 2007.

Baicker K and Goldman D, "Patient Cost-Sharing and Healthcare Spending Growth," *Journal of Economic Perspectives*, Vol. 25, No. 2, Spring 2011, pp. 47–68.

Barbash GI and Glied SA, "New Technology and Health Care Costs—The Case of Robot-Assisted Surgery," *New England Journal of Medicine*, Vol. 363, No. 8, August 19, 2010, pp. 701–704.

Bentley TGK, Effros R, Palar K, and Keeler EB, "Waste in the U.S. Health Care System: A Conceptual Framework," *The Milbank Quarterly*, Vol. 86, No. 4, December 2008, pp. 629–659.

Berwick DM, "Launching Accountable Care Organizations—The Proposed Rule for the Medicare Shared Savings Program," *New England Journal of Medicine*, Vol. 364, No. 16, April 21, 2011, p. e32.

Bishop TF, Federman AD, and Keyhani S, "Physicians' Views on Defensive Medicine: A National Survey," *Archives of Internal Medicine*, Vol. 170, No. 12, June 28, 2010, pp. 1081–1083.

Blume-Kohout ME, "Does Targeted, Disease-Specific Public Research Funding Influence Pharmaceutical Innovation?" *Journal of Policy Analysis and Management*, Vol. 31, No. 3, Summer 2012, pp. 641–660.

Brennan RA, Bodenheimer T, and Pham HH, "Specialty Service Lines: Salvos in the New Medical Arms Race," *Health Affairs*, Vol. 25, No. 5, September–October 2006, pp. w337–w343.

Brennan TJ, Maccauley MK, and Whitefoot KS, *Prizes or Patents for Technology Development—An Assessment and Analytic Framework*, discussion paper DP 11-21-REV, Washington D.C.: Resources for the Future, December 2012.

Brenner DJ and Hall EJ, "Computed Tomography—An Increasing Source of Radiation Exposure," *New England Journal of Medicine*, Vol. 357, November 29, 2007, pp. 2277–2284.

Brill S, "Bitter Pill: Why Medical Bills Are Killing Us," *Time*, February 20, 2013.

Brown SH, Lincoln MJ, Groen PJ, and Kolodner RM, "VistA—U.S. Department of Veterans Affairs National-Scale HIS," *International Journal of Medical Informatics*, Vol. 69, No. 2–3, March 2003, pp. 135–156.

Buntin MB, Haviland AM, McDevitt R, and Sood N, "Healthcare Spending and Preventive Care in High-Deductible and Consumer-Directed Health Plans," *American Journal of Managed Care*, Vol. 17, No. 3, March 2011, pp. 222–230.

Buxton MJ and Chambers JD, "What Values Do the Public Want Their Health Systems to Use in Evaluating Technologies?" *European Journal of Health Economics*, Vol. 12, No. 4, August 2011, pp. 285–288.

Calfee JE, Berndt ER, Hahn R, Philipson T, Rubin P, and Viscusi WK, "Brief of John E. Calfee, Ernst R. Berndt, Robert Hahn, Tomas Philipson, Paul Rubin, and W. Kip Viscusi as *Amici Curiae* Supporting Petitioner" (in *Wyeth v. Levine*)," June 3, 2008.

Camarillo DB, Krummel TM, and Salisbury JK Jr, "Robotic Technology in Surgery: Past, Present, and Future," *American Journal of Surgery*, Vol. 188, Supplement 4A, October 2004, pp. 2S–15S.

Carnahan SJ, "Medicare's Coverage with Study Participation: Clinical Trials or Tribulations?" *Yale Journal of Health Policy, Law, and Ethics*, Vol. 7, No. 2, Summer 2007, pp. 230–272.

Carrier E, Pham HH, and Rich EC, *Comparative Effectiveness Research and Innovation: Policy Options to Foster Medical Advances*, National Institute for Health Care Reform (NIHCR), NIHCR Policy Analysis No. 3, October 2010.

Carrns A, "Trends to Watch for in Employer Health Plans," *New York Times*, September 26, 2013. As of February 16, 2014:
http://www.nytimes.com/2013/09/26/your-money/
trends-to-watch-for-in-employer-health-plans.html?_r=0&pagewanted=print

Cassel CK and Guest JA, "Choosing Wisely—Helping Physicians and Patients Make Smart Decisions About Their Care," *Journal of the American Medical Association*, Vol. 307, No. 17, May 2, 2012, pp. 1801–1802.

Centers for Disease Control and Prevention, "Achievements in Public Health, 1900–1999: Impact of Vaccines Universally Recommended for Children—United States, 1990–1998," *Morbidity and Mortality Weekly*, Vol. 48, No. 12, April 2, 1999a, pp. 243–248. As of January 7, 2014: http://www.cdc.gov/mmwr/preview/mmwrhtml/00056803.htm

Centers for Disease Control and Prevention, "Ten Great Public Health Achievements—United States, 1900–1999," *Morbidity and Mortality Weekly*, Vol. 48, No. 12, April 2, 1999b, pp. 241–243. As of January 7, 2014: http://www.cdc.gov/mmwr/preview/mmwrhtml/00056796.htm

Centers for Medicare & Medicaid Services, "Innovation Models," undated (a). As of March 10, 2014: http://innovation.cms.gov/initiatives/#views=models

Centers for Medicare & Medicaid Services, National Health Expenditures 2012 Highlights, undated (b).

Centers for Medicare & Medicaid Services, *Hospital Outpatient Prospective Payment System*, Payment System Fact Sheet Series, ICN 006820, December 2012.

Centers for Medicare & Medicaid Services, "Medicare Dashboard Advances ACA Goals for Chronic Conditions," press release, March 28, 2013a. As of December 30, 2013: http://www.cms.gov/Newsroom/MediaReleaseDatabase/Press-Releases/2013-Press-Releases-Items/2013-03-28.html

Centers for Medicare & Medicaid Services, *Chronic Conditions Among Medicare Beneficiaries—Chartbook: 2012 Edition*, April 25, 2013b. As of December 30, 2013: http://www.cms.gov/Research-Statistics-Data-and-Systems/Statistics-Trends-and-Reports/Chronic-Conditions/2012ChartBook.html

Centers for Medicare & Medicaid Services, "Qualified Electronic Health Record (EHR) Direct Vendors for the 2013 Physician Quality Reporting System (PQRS) and Electronic Prescribing (eRx) Incentive Programs," August 21, 2013c. As of February 11, 2014: http://www.cms.gov/Medicare/Quality-Initiatives-Patient-Assessment-Instruments/PQRS/Downloads/2013QualifiedEHRDirectVendors.pdf

Chambers JD, "Medicare Coverage Decision Emphasizes CMS-FDA Coordination," Cost-Effectiveness Analysis Registry, The CEA Registry Blog, February 23, 2012. As of February 13, 2014: https://research.tufts-nemc.org/cear4/Resources/CEARegistryBlog/tabid/69/EntryId/198/Medicare-coverage-decision-emphasizes-CMS-FDA-coordination.aspx

Chambers JD, Neumann PJ, and Buxton MJ, "Does Medicare Have an Implicit Cost-Effectiveness Threshold?" *Medical Decision Making*, Vol. 30, No. 4, June 15, 2010, pp. E14–E27.

Chandra A, Cutler D, and Song Z, "Who Ordered That? The Economics of Treatment Choices in Medical Care," Chapter Six in Pauly MV, Mcguire TG, and Barros PB, eds., *Handbook of Health Economics*, Vol. 2, 2012, pp. 397–432.

Chandra A and J Skinner, "Technology Growth and Expenditure Growth in Health Care," *Journal of Economic Literature*, Vol. 50, No. 3, September 2012, pp. 645–680.

Chatterji AK, "Spawned with a Silver Spoon? Entrepreneurial Performance and Innovation in the Medical Device Industry," *Strategic Management Journal*, Vol. 30, No. 2, February 2008, pp. 185–206.

Chernew ME, Juster IA, Shah M, Wegh A, Rosenberg S, Rosen AB, Sokol MC, Yu-Isenberg K, and Fendrick AM, "Evidence That Value-Based Insurance Can Be Effective," *Health Affairs,* Vol. 29, No. 3, March 2010, pp. 530–536.

Chernew ME and Newhouse JP, "Health Care Spending Growth," Chapter One in Pauly MV, Mcguire TG, and Barros PB, eds., *Handbook of Health Economics*, Vol. 2, 2012, pp. 1–43.

Chernew ME, Rosen AB, and Fendrick AM, "Value-Based Insurance Design," *Health Affairs,* Vol. 26, No. 2, March 2007, pp. w195–w203.

Choosing Wisely, home page, 2014. As of March 15, 2014:
http://www.choosingwisely.org/

CMS—*see* Centers for Medicare & Medicaid Services.

Cohen JT, Neumann PJ, and Weinstein MC, "Does Preventive Care Save Money? Health Economics and the Presidential Candidates," *New England Journal of Medicine*, Vol. 387, No. 7, February 14, 2008, pp. 661–663.

CommonWell Health Alliance, home page, 2014. As of March 17, 2014:
http://www.commonwellalliance.org

Congressional Budget Office, *Research and Development in the Pharmaceutical Industry*, Washington, D.C., 2006.

Congressional Budget Office, *Prescription Drug Pricing in the Private Sector*, Washington, D.C., 2007.

Congressional Budget Office, *Technological Change and the Growth of Health Care Spending*, Washington, D.C., January 2008. As of September 29, 2013:
http://www.cbo.gov/sites/default/files/cbofiles/ftpdocs/89xx/doc8947/01-31-techhealth.pdf

Congressional Budget Office, The 2013 Long-Term Budget Outlook, September 17, 2013. As of March 17, 2014:
http://www.cbo.gov/publication/44521

Coombs B, "The Race for Next-Generation Alzheimer's Drugs," CNBC, September 5, 2013. As of February 12, 2014:
http://www.cnbc.com/id/101011893

Cutler DM, *Your Money or Your Life: Strong Medicine for America's Health Care System*, Oxford University Press, 2004.

Cutler DM and McClellan M, "Is Technological Change in Medicine Worth It?" *Health Affairs,* Vol. 20, No. 5, September 2001, pp. 11–29.

Cutler DM, Rosen AB, and Vijan S, "The Value of Medical Spending in the United States, 1960–2000," *New England Journal of Medicine*, Vol. 355, August 31, 2006, pp. 920–927.

Cutler DM and Sahni NR, "If Slow Rate of Health Care Spending Growth Persists, Projections May Be Off by $770 Billion," *Health Affairs*, Vol. 32, No. 5, May 2013, pp. 841–850.

Daniel GW, Rubens EK, and McClellan M, "Coverage with Evidence Development for Medicare Beneficiaries—Challenges and Next Steps," *JAMA Internal Medicine*, Vol. 173, No. 14, July 22, 2013, pp. 1281–1282.

Devers KJ, Brewster LR, and Casalino LP, "Changes in Hospital Competitive Strategy: A New Medical Arms Race?" *Health Services Research*, Vol. 38, No. 1, Part 2, February 2003, pp. 447–469.

Dolan P, "The Measurement of Health-Related Quality of Life for Use in Resource Allocation Decisions in Health Care," in Culyer AJ and Newhouse J, eds., *Handbook of Health Economics*, Oxford: Elsevier, 2000, pp. 1723–1760.

Eastwood B, "Why Healthcare Providers Aren't Happy with EHR Systems," *CIO*, July 1, 2013. As of October 30, 2013:
http://www.cio.com/article/735754/
Why_Healthcare_Providers_Aren_t_Happy_With_EHR_Systems

Edney A and Larkin C, "Drug Approvals Reach 15-Year High on Smoother FDA Reviews," Bloomberg, January 1, 2013. As of November 5, 2013:
http://www.bloomberg.com/news/2013-01-02/
drug-approvals-reach-15-year-high-on-smoother-fda-reviews.html

Emanuel EJ, "A Plan to Fix Cancer Care," *New York Times*, Opinionator blog, March 23, 2013. As of October 31, 2013:
http://opinionator.blogs.nytimes.com/2013/03/23/a-plan-to-fix-cancer-care

Emanuel EJ and Person SD, "It Costs More, But Is It Worth More?" *New York Times*, January 2, 2012. As of January 30, 2014:
http://opinionator.blogs.nytimes.com/2012/01/02/it-costs-more-but-is-it-worth-more/?_r=0

Engelberg Center for Health Care Reform at Brookings, *Bending the Curve—Person-Centered Health Care Reform: A Framework for Improving Care and Slowing Health Care Cost Growth*, 2013. As of January 7, 2014:
http://www.brookings.edu/research/reports/2013/04/person-centered-health-care-reform#

Esserman LJ, Thompson IM, and Reid B, "Overdiagnosis and Overtreatment in Cancer: An Opportunity for Improvement," *Journal of the American Medical Association*, Vol. 310, No. 8, August 28, 2013, pp. 797–798.

Executive Office of the President, President's Council of Advisors on Science and Technology, *Realizing the Full Potential of Health Information Technology to Improve Healthcare for Americans: The Path Forward*, Report to the President, December 2010. As of October 28, 2013:
http://www.whitehouse.gov/sites/default/files/microsites/ostp/pcast-health-it-report.pdf

FamiliesUSA, "Medicaid," 2014. As of March 17, 2014:
http://familiesusa.org/issues/medicaid/

Fang FC and Casadevall A, "NIH Peer Review Reform—Change We Need or Lipstick on a Pig?" *Infection and Immunology*, Vol. 77, No. 3, March 2009, pp. 929–932.

FDA—*see* U.S. Food and Drug Administration.

Feifer AH, Elkin EB, Lowrance WT, Denton B, Jacks L, Yee DS, Coleman JA, Laudone VP, Scardino PT, and Eastham JA, "Temporal Trends and Predictors of Pelvic Lymph Node Dissection in Open or Minimally Invasive Radical Prostatectomy," *Cancer*, Vol. 117, No. 17, September 1, 2011, pp. 3933–3942.

Fendrick AM, Chernew M, and Levi GW, "Value-Based Insurance Design: Embracing Value Over Costs Alone," *American Journal of Managed Care*, Vol. 15, No. 10, Supplement, December 2009, pp. S277–S283.

Fendrick AM, Smith DG, and Chernew ME, "Applying Value-Based Insurance to Low-Value Health Services," *Health Affairs*, Vol. 29, No. 11, November 1, 2010, pp. 2017–2021.

Foote SB, "Focus on Locus: Evolution of Medicare's Local Coverage Policy," *Health Affairs*, Vol. 22, No. 4, July–August 2003, pp. 137–146.

Fuchs VR, "Major Trends in the U.S. Health Economy Since 1950," *New England Journal of Medicine*, Vol. 366, March 15, 2012, pp. 973–977. As of September 29, 2013:
http://www.nejm.org/doi/full/10.1056/NEJMp1200478

GAO—*see* U.S. Government Accountability Office.

Garber A, "Advances in Cost-Effectiveness Analysis," Chapter Four in Culyer AJ and Newhouse JP, eds., *Handbook of Health Economics*, Vol. 1, Part 1, Elsevier, 2000.

Garber AM, "Cost-Effectiveness and Evidence Evaluation as Criteria for Coverage Policy," *Health Affairs*, May 19, 2004, pp. W4, 284–296.

Garber AM and Skinner J, "Is American Health Care Uniquely Inefficient?" *Journal of Economic Perspectives*, Vol. 22, No. 4, Fall 2008, pp. 27–50.

Garber A and Sox HC, "The Role of Costs in Comparative Effectiveness Research," *Health Affairs*, Vol. 29, No. 10, October 2010, pp. 1805–1811.

Garber S, *Economic Effects of Product Liability and Other Litigation Involving the Safety and Effectiveness of Pharmaceuticals,* Santa Monica, Calif.: RAND Corporation, MG-1259-ICJ, 2013. As of September 29, 2013:
http://www.rand.org/pubs/monographs/MG1259.html

Garber S, Ridgely MS, Taylor R, and Meili R, *Managed Care and the Evaluation and Adoption of Emerging Medical Technologies*, Santa Monica, Calif.: RAND Corporation, MR-1195-HIMA, 2000. As of August 19, 2011:
http://www.rand.org/pubs/monograph_reports/MR1195.html

Gawande A, "Letting Go," *The New Yorker*, August 2, 2010. As of October 31, 2013:
http://www.newyorker.com/reporting/2010/08/02/100802fa_fact_gawande

Gawande A, "Big Med," *The New Yorker*, August 13, 2012. As of October 29, 2013:
http://www.newyorker.com/reporting/2012/08/13/120813fa_fact_gawande

Glassman E, Hanson WA, Kazanzides P, Mittelstadt BD, Musits BL, Paul HA, and Taylor RH, "Image-Directed Robotic System for Precise Robotic Surgery Including Redundant Consistency Checking," U.S. Patent US5086401 A, February 4, 1992.

Glennerster R and Kremer M, "A Better Way to Spur Medical Research and Development," *Regulation*, Vol. 23, No. 2, Summer 2000, pp. 34–39.

Gold J, "Proton Beam Therapy Heats Up Hospital Arms Race," Kaiser Health News, May 31, 2013.

Gold MR, Siegel JE, Russell LB, and Weinstein MC, eds., *Cost-Effectiveness in Health and Medicine*, New York: Oxford University Press, 1996.

Goldman D and Lakdawalla D, "Intellectual Property, Information Technology, Biomedical Research, and Marketing of Patented Products," in *Handbook of Health Economics*, Vol. 2, 2012.

Grabowski HG and Vernon JM, *The Regulation of Pharmaceuticals: Balancing the Benefits and Risks*, American Enterprise Institute for Public Policy Research, 1983.

Graham SJH, Merges RP, Samuelson P, and Sichelman TM, "High Technology Entrepreneurs and the Patent System: Results of the 2008 Berkeley Patent Survey," unpublished manuscript, 2009.

Guell RC and Fischbaum M, "Toward Allocative Efficiency in the Prescription Drug Industry," *Milbank Quarterly*, Vol. 73, No. 2, 1995, pp. 213–230.

Hancock J, "Hospital CEO Bonuses Reward Volume and Growth," Kaiser Health News, June 16, 2013. As of October 31, 2013:
http://www.kaiserhealthnews.org/stories/2013/june/06/hospital-ceo-compensation-mainbar.aspx

Hanna KE, *Innovation and Invention in Medical Devices: Workshop Summary*, National Academies Press, 2001.

Hare J, Testimony to the House Committee on Ways and Means, Subcommittee on Health, Washington, D.C., July 20, 2010. As of November 1, 2013:
http://waysandmeans.house.gov/media/pdf/111/2010jul20_hare_testimony.pdf

Harrington SE, *Incentivizing Comparative Effectiveness Research*, The Wharton School, University of Pennsylvania, January 2011.

Haviland AM, Sood N, McDevitt RD, and Marquis MS, "The Effects of Consumer-Directed Health Plans on Episodes of Health Care," *Forum for Health Economics & Policy*, Vol. 14, No. 2, Article 9, September 2011.

"Health Policy Brief: Excise Tax on 'Cadillac' Plans," Health Affairs, September 12, 2013. As of February 16, 2014:
http://www.healthaffairs.org/healthpolicybriefs/brief.php?brief_id=99

Herper M, "Five Health IT Firms Band Together to Create a National System for Identifying Patients and Sharing Medical Records," *Forbes*, March 4, 2013. As of October 19, 2013:
http://www.forbes.com/sites/matthewherper/2013/03/04/
exclusive-health-it-firms-join-forces-to-create-national-system-for-sharing-medical-records/

HHMI—*see* Howard Hughes Medical Institute.

HHS—*see* U.S. Department of Health and Human Services.

Howard Hughes Medical Institute, "About Us," 2013. As of December 30, 2013:
http://www.hhmi.org/about

Hu JC, Gu X, Lipsitz SR, Barry MJ, D'Amico AV, Weinberg AC, and Keating NL, "Comparative Effectiveness of Minimally Invasive Vs. Open Radical Prostatectomy," *Journal of the American Medical Association*, Vol. 302, No. 14, October 14, 2009, pp. 1557–1564.

Hurwitz H, Fehrenbacher L, Novotny W, Cartwright T, Hainsworth J, Heim W, Berlin J, Baron A, Griffing S, Holmgren E, Ferrara N, Fyfe G, Rogers B, Ross R, and Kabbinavar F, "Bevacizumab Plus Irinotecan, Fluorouracil, and Leucovorin for Metastatic Colorectal Cancer," *New England Journal of Medicine*, Vol. 350, No. 23, June 3, 2004, pp. 2335–2342.

IMS Health, "Top-Line Market Data," 2014. As of February 11, 2014:
http://www.imshealth.com/portal/site/ims/menuitem.5ad1c081663fdf9b41d84b903208c22a/
?vgnextoid=fbc65890d33ee210VgnVCM10000071812ca2RCRD

Institute of Medicine, *U.S. Health in International Perspective: Shorter Lives, Poorer Health*, National Academies Press, January 9, 2013. As of November 1, 2013:
http://www.iom.edu/Reports/2013/
US-Health-in-International-Perspective-Shorter-Lives-Poorer-Health.aspx

IOM—*see* Institute of Medicine.

Kaiser Family Foundation, "Medicare Spending and Financing Fact Sheet," November 14, 2012. As of January 2, 2014:
http://kff.org/medicare/fact-sheet/medicare-spending-and-financing-fact-sheet/

Kaiser Family Foundation, "Assessing the Effects of the Economy on the Recent Slowdown in Health Spending," Issue Brief, April 22, 2013. As of October 31, 2013:
http://kff.org/health-costs/issue-brief/
assessing-the-effects-of-the-economy-on-the-recent-slowdown-in-health-spending-2/

Kaiser Family Foundation and Health Research & Educational Trust, Employer Health Benefits, "2013 Summary of Findings," August 20, 2013. As of March 17, 2014:
http://kff.org/report-section/2013-summary-of-findings/

Keeler E, Melnick G, and Zwanziger J, "The Changing Effects of Competition on Non-Profit and For-Profit Hospital Pricing Behavior," *Journal of Health Economics*, Vol. 18, No. 1, January 1999, pp. 69–86.

Keller DM, "Proton Beam Radiation Therapy: The 'Chicken & Egg' Dilemma, Part 1 of a Multipart Investigation," *Oncology Times*, Vol. 32, No. 6, March 25, 2010a, pp. 35–36, 39–40.

Keller DM, "Proton Beam Radiation Therapy: The 'Chicken & Egg' Dilemma, Part 2, Continuing Series," *Oncology Times*, Vol. 32, No. 7, April 10, 2010b, pp. 35–36.

Kelley AS, Deb P, Du Q, Aldridge Carlson MD, and Morrison RS, "Hospice Enrollment Saves Money for Medicare snd Improves Care Quality Across a Number of Different Lengths-of-Stay," *Health Affairs*, Vol. 32, No. 3, March 2013, pp. 552–561.

Kesselheim AS, Myers JA, Solomon DH, Winkelmayer WC, Levin R, and Avorn J, "The Prevalence and Cost of Unapproved Uses of Top-Selling Orphan Drugs," *PLoS ONE*, Vol. 7, No. 2, February 21, 2012.

Ketcham JD and Furukawa MF, "Hospital-Physician Gainsharing in Cardiology," *Health Affairs*, Vol. 27, No. 3, May 2008, pp. 803–812.

Kliff S, "Steven Brill's 26,000-Word Health-Care Story, in One Sentence," *Washington Post*, Wonkblog, February 23, 2013. As of October 28, 2013:
http://www.washingtonpost.com/blogs/wonkblog/wp/2013/02/23/
steven-brills-26000-word-health-care-story-in-one-sentence/

Knowledge Ecology International, "Annotated Bibliography of Articles and Books on Innovation Prizes," undated. As of December 26, 2013:
http://keionline.org/prizes/cites

Knowledge Ecology International, *Selected Innovation Prizes and Reward Programs*, KEI Research Note No. 2008:1, 2008.

Kocher R and Roberts B, "The Calculus of Cures," *New England Journal of Medicine*, published online February 26, 2014.

Kolata G, "FDA Plans Looser Rules on Approving Alzheimer's Drugs," *New York Times*, March 13, 2013. As of February 12, 2014:
http://www.nytimes.com/2013/03/14/health/fda-to-ease-alzheimers-drug-approval-rules.html?_r=0

Korobkin R, *Relative Value Health Insurance: A Behavioral Law and Economics Solution to the Medical Care Cost Crises*, UCLA Law & Economics Series, 2012. As of September 29, 2013:
http://escholarship.org/uc/item/6j85h1dc

Kozauer N and Katz R, "Regulatory Innovation and Drug Development for Early-Stage Alzheimer's Disease," *New England Journal of Medicine*, Vol. 368, March 28, 2013, pp. 1169–1171.

Kremer M, "Patent Buyouts: A Mechanism for Encouraging Innovation," *Quarterly Journal of Economics*, Vol. 113, No. 4, November 1998, pp. 1137–1167.

Kulkarni SS, "Quick Facts About High-Deductible Health Plans," Kaiser Health News, April 27, 2012. As of March 17, 2014:
http://www.kaiserhealthnews.org/stories/2012/april/27/high-deductible-health-plans.aspx

Lakhani KR and Jeppesen LB, "Getting Unusual Suspects to Solve R&D Puzzles," *Harvard Business Review*, May 2007, pp. 30, 32.

Lakhani KR, Jeppesen LB, Lohse PA, and Panetta JA, "The Value of Openness in Scientific Problem Solving," Discussion Paper 07-050, Harvard Business School, October 2006.

Lee J, "FDA to Offer Draft Guidance on Interoperability of Medical Devices," *Modern Healthcare*, February 6, 2014. As of February 12, 2014:
http://www.modernhealthcare.com/article/20140206/NEWS/302069934

Levey NN, "Doctors List Overused Medical Treatments," *Los Angeles Times*, February 20, 2013. As of December 29, 2013:
http://articles.latimes.com/2013/feb/20/nation/la-na-medical-procedures-20130221

Lo Sasso AT, Helmchen L, and Kaestner R, "The Effects of Consumer-Directed Health Plans on Health Care Spending," *Journal of Risk and Insurance*, Vol. 77, No. 1, March 2010, pp. 85–103.

Luft HS, "Economic Incentives to Promote Innovation in Healthcare Delivery," *Clinical Orthopaedics and Related Research*, online exclusive, June 19, 2009.

Mack MJ, "Minimally Invasive and Robotic Surgery," *Journal of the American Medical Association*, Vol. 285, No. 5, February 7, 2001, pp. 568–572.

Makower J, Meer A, and Denend L, *FDA Impact on U.S. Medical Technology Innovation: A Survey of Over 200 Medical Technology Companies*, November 2010.

Marshall JL, Cheson BD, and Kerr D, "Physicians 'Hit the Barricades' Over Cancer Costs," *Medscape Oncology*, June 10, 2013. As of October 21, 2013:
http://www.medscape.com/viewarticle/805503

Matthews CA, "The Promise of Robotics in Urogynecology," *International Urogynecology Journal*, Vol. 23, No. 9, September 2012, pp. 1177–1178.

McClellan MB and Tunis SR, "Medicare Coverage of ICDs," *New England Journal of Medicine*, Vol. 352, No. 3, January 20, 2005, pp. 222–224.

Medicaid.gov, "Managed Care," undated. As of February 6, 2014:
http://www.medicaid.gov/Medicaid-CHIP-Program-Information/By-Topics/Delivery-Systems/Managed-Care/Managed-Care.html

Mello MM, Studdert DM, and Brennan TA, "Shifting Terrain in the Regulation of Off-Label Promotion of Pharmaceuticals," *New England Journal of Medicine*, Vol. 360, No. 15, April 9, 2009, pp. 1557–1566.

Melnick G and Keeler E, "The Effects of Multi-Hospital Systems on Hospital Prices," *Journal of Health Economics*, Vol. 26, No. 2, March 1, 2007, pp. 400–413.

Meltzer DO and Smith P, "Theoretical Issues Relevant to the Economic Evaluation of Health Technologies," Chapter Seven in Culyer AJ, Pauly MV, Newhouse JP, McGuire TG, and Barros PP, eds., *Handbook of Health Economics*, Vol. 2, Elsevier, 2012, pp. 433–470.

Miller K, Wang M, Gralow J, Dickler M, Cobleigh M, Perez EA, Shenkier T, Cella D, and Davidson NE, "Paclitaxel Plus Bevacizumab Versus Paclitaxel Alone for Metastatic Breast Cancer," *New England Journal of Medicine*, Vol. 357, No. 26, December 27, 2007, pp. 2666–2676.

Morgan S, Grootendorst P, Lexchin J, Cunningham C, and Greyson D, "The Cost of Drug Development: A Systematic Review," *Health Policy*, Vol. 100, No. 1, April 2011, pp. 4–17.

Moukheiber Z, "An Interview with the Most Powerful Woman in Health Care," *Forbes*, May 15, 2013.

Moussa, Nader (Nimur), "Laproscopic Surgery Robot," 2004. As of March 28, 2014:
http://en.wikipedia.org/wiki/File:Laproscopic_Surgery_Robot.jpg

Murray K, "How Doctors Die—It's Not Like the Rest of Us, But It Should Be," Zócalo Public Square, November 30, 2011. As of December 30, 2013:
http://www.zocalopublicsquare.org/2011/11/30/how-doctors-die/ideas/nexus/

Murray K, "Doctors Really Do Die Differently," Zócalo Public Square, July 23, 2012. As of December 30, 2013:
http://www.zocalopublicsquare.org/2012/07/23/doctors-really-do-die-differently/ideas/nexus/

National Association for Proton Therapy, home page, 2013. As of November 5, 2013:
http://www.proton-therapy.org

National Cancer Institute, "FDA Approval for Bevacizumab," updated July 1, 2013. As of January 10, 2014:
http://www.cancer.gov/cancertopics/druginfo/fda-bevacizumab

National Heart, Lung, and Blood Institute, "What Is an Implantable Cardioverter Defibrillator?" revised August 2009. As of March 25, 2014:
http://www.nhlbi.nih.gov/health//dci/images/scd_icd.jpg

National Institutes of Health, "NIH Budget" September 18, 2012. As of December 30, 2013:
http://www.nih.gov/about/budget.htm

National Institutes of Health, "High-Risk Research—Overview," June 26, 2013a. As of December 30, 2013:
https://commonfund.nih.gov/highrisk/overview

National Institutes of Health, "NIH Announces 2013 High-Risk, High-Reward Research Awards," September 30, 2013b. As of December 30, 2013:
http://www.nih.gov/news/health/sep2013/od-30.htm

National Institutes of Health, Office of Budget, "Spending History by Institute/Center, Mechanism, Etc. (1983 to present)," 2013. As of November 5, 2013:
http://officeofbudget.od.nih.gov/spending_hist.html

National Institutes of Health, Office of Extramural Research, "Qualifying Therapeutic Discovery Project Program," June 18, 2010. As of March 17, 2014:
http://grants.nih.gov/grants/funding/QTDP_PIM/

Neumann PJ and Chambers JD, "Medicare's Enduring Struggle to Define 'Reasonable and Necessary' Care," *New England Journal of Medicine*, November 8, 2012, pp. 1775–1777.

Neumann PJ and Chambers J, "Medicare's Reset on 'Coverage with Evidence Development,'" Health Affairs Blog, April 1, 2013. As of January 4, 2013:
http://healthaffairs.org/blog/2013/04/01/medicares-reset-on-coverage-with-evidence-development/

Neumann PJ, Divi N, Beinfeld MT, Levine BS, Keenan PS, Halpern EF, and Gazelle GS, "Medicare's National Coverage Decisions, 1999–2003: Quality of Evidence and Review," *Health Affairs*, Vol. 24, No. 1, 2005, pp. 243–254.

Neumann PJ, Kamae MS, and Palmer JA, "Medicare's National Coverage Decisions for Technologies, 1999–2007," *Health Affairs*, Vol. 27, No. 6, November–December 2008, pp. 1620–1631.

Newhouse JP, "Why Is There a Quality Chasm?" *Health Affairs*, Vol. 21, No. 4, July 2002, pp. 13–25. As of September 29, 2013:
http://content.healthaffairs.org/content/21/4/13.full

Newhouse JP and the Insurance Experiment Group, *Free for All? Lessons from the RAND Health Insurance Experiment*, Cambridge, Mass.: Harvard University Press, CB-199, 1993. As of October 31, 2013:
http://www.rand.org/pubs/commercial_books/CB199.html

NIH—*see* National Institutes of Health.

Orenstein P, "Our Feel-Good War on Breast Cancer," *New York Times*, April 25, 2013. As of October 31, 2013:
http://www.nytimes.com/2013/04/28/magazine/our-feel-good-war-on-breast-cancer.html?_r=0

Orszag P, "How Health Care Can Save or Sink America: The Case for Reform and Fiscal Sustainability," *Foreign Affairs*, Vol. 90, No. 4, July/August 2011, pp. 42–57.

Patient-Centered Outcomes Research Institute, "Research We Support," 2014. As of March 10, 2014: http://www.pcori.org/research-we-support/landing/

PCORI—*see* Patient-Centered Outcomes Research Institute.

Pearson SD and Bach PB, "How Medicare Could Use Comparative Effectiveness Research in Deciding on New Coverage and Reimbursement," *Health Affairs*, Vol. 29, No. 10, October 2010, pp. 1796–1804.

Peltola H, "Worldwide Haemophilus influenzae Type b Disease at the Beginning of the 21st Century: Global Analysis of the Disease Burden 25 Years After the Use of the Polysaccharide Vaccine and a Decade After the Advent of Conjugates," *Clinical Microbiology Reviews*, Vol. 13, No. 2, April 2000, pp. 302–317.

Peltzman S, *Regulation of Pharmaceutical Innovation: The 1962 Amendments (Evaluative Studies 15)*, American Enterprise Institute for Public Policy Research, 1974.

Pham HH, Ginsburg PB, Lake TK, and Maxwell MM, *Episode-Based Payments: Charting a Course for Health Care Payment Reform*, Washington, D.C.: National Institute for Health Care Reform, January 2010.

Pharmaceutical Research and Manufacturers of America (PhRMA), "Medicines in Development—Alzheimer's Disease," 2013.

Philipson T, Eber M, Lakdawalla DN, Corral M, Conti R, and Goldman DP, "Analysis of Whether Higher Health Care Spending in the United States Versus Europe Is 'Worth It' in the Case of Cancer," *Health Affairs*, Vol. 31, No. 4, April 2012, pp. 667–675.

Philipson TJ and Sun E, "Is the Food and Drug Administration Safe and Effective?" *Journal of Economic Perspectives*, Vol. 22, No. 1, 2008, pp. 85–102.

PhRMA—*see* Pharmaceutical Research and Manufacturers of America.

Pollack A, "Doctors Denounce Cancer Drug Prices of $100,000 a Year," *New York Times*, April 25, 2013. As of October 30, 2013:
http://www.nytimes.com/2013/04/26/business/cancer-physicians-attack-high-drug-costs.html

Pstay BM and Ray W, "FDA Guidance on Off-Label Promotion and the State of the Literature from Sponsors," *Journal of the American Medical Association*, Vol. 299, No. 16, April 23/30, 2008, pp. 1949–1951.

Radley DC, Finkelstein SN, and Stafford RS, "Off-Label Prescribing Among Office-Based Physicians," *Archives of Internal Medicine*, Vol. 166, No. 9, May 8, 2006, pp. 1021–1026.

Robbins CJ, Rudsenske T, and Vaughan JS, "Private Equity Investments in Health Care," *Health Affairs*, Vol. 27, No. 5, September/October 2008, pp. 1389–1398.

Robinson JC, "Applying Value-Based Insurance Design to High-Cost Health Services," *Health Affairs*, Vol. 29, No. 11, November 2010, pp. 2009–2015.

Robinson JC, "Providers' Payment and Delivery System Reforms Hold Both Threats and Opportunities for the Drug and Device Industries," *Health Affairs*, Vol. 31, No. 9, September 2012, pp. 2059–2067.

Robinson JC and Luft HS, "Competition and the Cost of Hospital Care, 1972 to 1982," *Journal of the American Medical Association*, Vol. 257, No. 23, June 19, 1987, pp. 3241–3245.

Robinson JC and MacPherson K, "Payers Test Reference Pricing and Centers of Excellence to Steer Patients to Low-Price and High-Quality Providers," *Health Affairs*, Vol. 31, No. 9, September 2012, pp. 2028–2036.

Rosenberg T, "Prizes with an Eye Toward the Future," *New York Times*, Opinionator blog, February 29, 2012. As of January 5, 2014:
http://opinionator.blogs.nytimes.com/2012/02/29/prizes-with-an-eye-toward-the-future/?_r=0

Rosenberg T, "Revealing a Health Care Secret: The Price," *New York Times*, Opinionator blog, July 31, 2013. As of October 28, 2013:
http://opinionator.blogs.nytimes.com/2013/07/31/a-new-health-care-approach-dont-hide-the-price/

Rosenthal ET, "Proton Beam Radiation Therapy: Balancing Evidence-Based Use with the Bottom Line, Part 3 of a Series," *Oncology Times*, Vol. 32, No. 8, April 25, 2010a, pp. 34–38.

Rosenthal ET, "Proton Beam Radiation Therapy: Balancing Evidence-Based Use with the Bottom Line, Part 4 of a Series," *Oncology Times*, Vol. 32, No. 9, May 10, 2010b, pp. 28–30.

Rosenthal ET, "Proton Beam Radiation Therapy: The Case of Hampton University Proton Therapy Institute, Part 5 of a Series," *Oncology Times*, Vol. 32, No. 10, May 25, 2010c, pp. 26, 28–29.

Rosenthal E, "The Soaring Cost of a Simple Breath," *New York Times*, October 12, 2013. As of October 29, 2013:
http://www.nytimes.com/2013/10/13/us/the-soaring-cost-of-a-simple-breath.html

Rundle R, "In the Drive to Mine Medical Data, VHA Is the Unlikely Leader," *Wall Street Journal*, 2001, p. 1.

Russell LB, "Preventing Chronic Disease: An Important Investment, But Don't Count on Cost Savings," *Health Affairs*, Vol. 28, No. 1, January/February 2009, pp. 42–45.

Ryu AJ, Gibson TB, McKellar MR, and Chernew ME, "The Slowdown in Health Care Spending in 2009–11 Reflected Factors Other Than the Weak Economy and Thus May Persist," *Health Affairs*, Vol. 32, No. 5, May 2013, pp. 835–840.

Schleifer D and Rothman DJ, "'The Ultimate Decision Is Yours': Exploring Patients' Attitudes About the Overuse of Medical Interventions," *PLoS ONE*, Vol. 7, No. 12, December 2012, e52552. As of October 27, 2013:
http://www.plosone.org/article/info%3Adoi%2F10.1371%2Fjournal.pone.0052552

Schoen C, Guterman S, Shih A, Lau J, Kasimow S, Gauthier A, and Davis K, *Bending the Curve: Options for Achieving Savings and Improving Value in U.S. Health Spending*, Commonwealth Fund, December 2007. As of January 7, 2014:
http://www.commonwealthfund.org/Publications/Fund-Reports/2007/Dec/
Bending-the-Curve--Options-for-Achieving-Savings-and-Improving-Value-in-U-S--Health-Spending.
aspx

Scott Morton F and Kyle M, "Markets for Pharmaceutical Products," in Pauly MV, McGuire TG, and Barros PP, eds., *Handbook of Health Economics*, North Holland, 2012.

Sethi MK, Obremskey WT, Natividad H, Mir HR, and Jahangir AA, "Incidence and Costs of Defensive Medicine," *American Journal of Orthopedics*, Vol. 41, No. 2, February 2012, pp. 69–73.

Sloan FA, ed., *Valuing Health Care: Costs, Benefits, and Effectiveness of Pharmaceuticals and Other Medical Technologies*, Cambridge University Press, 1996.

Sloan FA and Shadle JH, "Is There Empirical Evidence for 'Defensive Medicine'? A Reassessment," *Journal of Health Economics*, Vol. 28, No. 2, March 2009, pp. 481–491.

Smith S, Newhouse JP, and Freeland MS, "Income, Insurance, and Technology: Why Does Health Spending Outpace Economic Growth?" *Health Affairs*, Vol. 28, No. 5, September/October 2009, pp. 1276–1284.

Sorenson C, Drummond M, and Khan BB, "Medical Technology as a Key Driver of Rising Health Expenditure: Disentangling the Relationship," *ClinicoEconomics and Outcomes Research*, Vol. 5, May 2013, pp. 223–234.

Sox HC, "Evaluating Off-Label Uses of Anticancer Drugs: Time for a Change," editorial, *Annals of Internal Medicine*, Vol. 150, No. 5, March 3, 2009, pp. 353–354.

Spurling GK, Mansfield PR, Montgomery BD, Lexchin J, Doust J, Othman N, and Vitry AI, "Information from Pharmaceutical Companies and the Quality, Quantity, and Cost of Physicians' Prescribing: A Systematic Review," *PLoS Medicine*, Vol. 7, No. 10, 2010.

Stafford RS, "Regulating Off-Label Drug Use: Rethinking the Role of the FDA," *New England Journal of Medicine*, Vol. 358, No. 14, 2008, pp. 1427–1429.

Stiglitz JE and Jayadev A, "Medicine for Tomorrow: Some Alternative Proposals to Promote Socially Beneficial Research and Development in Pharmaceuticals," *Journal of Generic Medicines: The Business Journal for the Generic Medicines Sector*, Vol. 7, No. 3, July 2010, pp. 217–226.

Stitzenberg KB, Wong YN, Nielsen ME, Egleston BL, and Uzzo RG, "Trends in Radical Prostatectomy: Centralization, Robotics, and Access to Urologic Cancer Care," *Cancer*, Vol. 118, No. 1, January 1, 2012, pp. 54–62.

Studdert DM, Mello MM, Sage WM, DesRoches CM, Peugh J, Zapert K and Brennan TA, "Defensive Medicine Among High-Risk Specialist Physicians in a Volatile Malpractice Environment," *Journal of the American Medical Association*, Vol. 293, No. 21, June 1, 2005, pp. 2609–2617.

Su LM, "Robot-Assisted Radical Prostatectomy: Advances Since 2005," *Current Opinion in Urology*, Vol. 20, No. 2, March 2010, pp. 130–135.

Thomas JW, Ziller EC, and Thayer DA, "Low Costs of Defensive Medicine, Small Savings from Tort Reform," *Health Affairs*, Vol. 29, No. 9, September 2010, pp. 1578–1584.

Tillman K, Burton B, Jacques LB, and Phurrough SE, "Compendia and Anticancer Therapy Under Medicare," *Annals of Internal Medicine*, Vol. 150, No. 5, March 3, 2009, pp. 348–350.

Toole AA, "Does Public Scientific Research Complement Private Research and Development Investment in the Pharmaceutical Industry?" *Journal of Law and Economics*, Vol. 50, No. 1, February 2007.

Tufts Center for the Study of Drug Development, "Biotech Products in Big Pharma Clinical Pipelines Have Grown Dramatically," news release, Boston, Mass., November 14, 2013. As of January 3, 2014:
http://csdd.tufts.edu/news/complete_story/pr_ir_nov_dec_2013

Tunis SR and Pearson SD, "Coverage Options for Promising Technologies: Medicare's 'Coverage with Evidence Development,'" *Health Affairs*, Vol. 25, No. 5, September–October 2006, pp. 1218–1230.

U.S. Department of Health and Human Services, "Doctors and Hospitals' Use of Health IT More Than Doubles Since 2012," news release, May 22, 2013. As of February 12, 2014:
http://www.hhs.gov/news/press/2013pres/05/20130522a.html

U.S. Food and Drug Administration, "Innovation Pathway," April 12, 2012. As of January 6, 2014:
http://www.fda.gov/AboutFDA/CentersOffices/OfficeofMedicalProductsandTobacco/CDRH/
CDRHInnovation/InnovationPathway/default.htm

U.S. Food and Drug Administration, "Fast Track, Breakthrough Therapy, Accelerated Approval and Priority Review," last updated June 26, 2013a. As of December 27, 2013:
http://www.fda.gov/forconsumers/byaudience/forpatientadvocates/
speedingaccesstoimportantnewtherapies/ucm128291.htm

U.S. Food and Drug Administration, "Medical Devices—Health IT Regulatory Framework," last updated September 11, 2013b. As of February 11, 2014:
http://www.fda.gov/MedicalDevices/ProductsandMedicalProcedures/ConnectedHealth/
ucm338920.htm

U.S. Food and Drug Administration, "FDA-CMS Parallel Review," last updated January 16, 2014. As of February 13, 2014:
http://www.fda.gov/MedicalDevices/DeviceRegulationandGuidance/HowtoMarketYourDevice/
PremarketSubmissions/ucm255678.htm

U.S. Government Accountability Office, *Medicare—Lack of Price Transparency May Hamper Hospitals' Ability to Be Prudent Purchasers of Implantable Medical Devices*, Washington, D.C., GAO-12-126, January 13, 2012a. As of October 27, 2013:
http://www.gao.gov/products/GAO-12-126

U.S. Government Accountability Office, *Medical Devices—FDA Has Met Most Performance Goals but Device Reviews Are Taking Longer*, Washington, D.C., GAO-12-418, February 29, 2012b. As of October 30, 2013:
http://www.gao.gov/products/GAO-12-418

U.S. Government Accountability Office, *Prescription Drugs—FDA Has Met Most Performance Goals for Reviewing Applications*, Washington, D.C., GAO-12-500, March 2012c. As of October 30, 2013:
http://www.gao.gov/products/GAO-12-500

University of Michigan Center for Value-Based Insurance Design, "The Evidence for V-BID: Validating an Intuitive Concept," V-BID Center Brief, Ann Arbor. Mich.: University of Michigan, November 2012. As of January 1, 2014:
http://www.sph.umich.edu/vbidcenter/publications/pdfs/
V-BID%20brief%20Evidence%20Nov2012.pdf

University of Michigan Center for Value-Based Insurance Design, "V-BID in Action: Driving Value Through Clinically Nuanced Incentives," V-BID Center Brief, Ann Arbor, Mich.: University of Michigan, February 2013. As of October 31, 2013:
http://www.sph.umich.edu/vbidcenter/publications/pdfs/
V-BID%20brief%20low-value%20Feb2013%20final.pdf

UpToDate, home page, 2014. As of March 17, 2014:
http://www.uptodate.com/home

Vernon JA, Golec JH, Lutter R, and Nardinelli C, "An Exploratory Study of FDA New Drug Review Times, Prescription Drug User Fee Acts, and R&D Spending," *Quarterly Review of Economics and Finance*, Vol. 49, No. 4, November 2009, pp. 1260–1274.

Weeks JC, Catalano PJ, Cronin A, Finkelman MD, Mack JW, Keating NL, and Schrag D, "Patients' Expectations About Effects of Chemotherapy for Advanced Cancer," *New England Journal of Medicine*, Vol. 367, October 25, 2012, pp. 1616–1625.

Wharam JF, Ross-Degnan D, and Rosenthal MB, "The ACA and High-Deductible Insurance—Strategies for Sharpening a Blunt Instrument," *New England Journal of Medicine*, Vol. 369, No. 16, October 17, 2013, pp. 1481–1484.

Zenios S, Makower J, and Yock P, eds., *Biodesign—The Process of Innovating Medical Technologies*, Cambridge, UK: Cambridge University Press, 2010.

Zhao D and Liu D, "Clinical Training Technology for Vascular Interventional Surgery Robot System Based on Master-Slave Expansion," 2012 International Conference on Mechatronics and Automation (ICMA), *Institute of Electrical and Electronics Engineers (IEEE)*, 2012, pp. 604–610.